The Recompense of a Great Reward That's Worth Dying For

A Christian Devotional
by
Dr. Ansley N. Mathis

He will wipe every tear from their eyes. There will
be no more death or mourning or crying or pain, for
the old order of things has passed away.
—Revelation 21:4

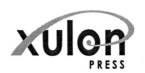

PRESS

Dedication & Acknowledgement

This book is dedicated to Jesus Christ (YaHshua)
unto the glory of God the Father YHWH Elohim.

This book is also dedicated to my husband and to
my mother.

Special thanks to the editor: Shae Cooke.

CONTENTS

PART 8: THE LAST CRY

Introduction

The cross was the instrument God chose for the redemption of mankind. Jesus refers to the hardships and sufferings of daily life as the "cross" that we must bear and embrace if we are to be His disciples and if we are to glorify the Father. Enduring these hardships for the sake of Christ gives our suffering a redeeming power and value—a share in the fruit—the recompense—the reward. Jesus more than anyone, suffered for His single-minded commitment to glorify God and bring about salvation. He was spit upon, whipped, bound, deceived, betrayed, falsely accused, struck, mocked, blasphemed, stripped, reviled, sneered at, smitten, bruised, chastised, wounded, cut off from the land of the living, and He hung on a cross for six agonizing hours. Yet He suffered for the sake of righteousness, to bring us to God, and to be our High Priest. However, evangelistic messages rarely focus on suffering as a necessary feature of Christianity. The emphasis is to lay it all at the cross—and the "carrying the cross" part comes much later, if at all, because some teach that if our faith is strong enough, we needn't suffer. However, this mindset not only fails to eliminate suffering, it robs believers of earthly and eternal rewards. An honest reading of Scripture reveals the inescapable truth that suffering is a prerequisite of our citizenship in heaven as residents of Earth. Jesus suffered and we know He didn't lack faith. Paul suffered not for a lack of faith, but for his faith. It's hard to see or sense the logic in suffering, especially the suffering of God's people, His church and His own Son, except, however, that the reward—the "recompense" makes it worthwhile!

In fact, Moses chose suffering for Christ over sinful pleasures "esteeming the reproach of Christ greater riches than the treasures in Egypt: for he had respect unto the recompense of the reward" (Hebrews 11:26). The saints who suffered for their faithful witness to Christ (at Smyrna) received this promise: "be thou faithful unto death, and I will give thee a crown of life" (Revelation 2:10b). We too will be recompensed for our perseverance, our suffering, and our faithful witness to Christ.

Believers are told, "The righteous shall be recompensed in the earth" (Proverbs. 11:31) and promised, "Behold, thy salvation cometh; behold, his reward is with him, and his work before him" (Isaiah 62:11b). Suffering is a real, and crucial, inescapable part of the Christian faith. It makes sense only in light of the promise of a great recompense of reward for our suffering. This is a recompense that makes it all worthwhile.

Of course, it's human nature not to like pain. Jesus' human nature shrank from pain just as our does. We see that in the Garden of Gethsemane, yet Jesus willingly accepted it when commanded by His Heavenly Father. The same should be true of us. When we accept suffering, we have the Father and the "Helper" to help us through it, as Jesus did. "For even hereunto were ye called: because Christ also suffered for us, leaving us an example, that ye should follow his steps" (1 Peter 2:21). We can pray in our gardens and ask God to let the cup of suffering pass from us, but if we're willing to let His will be done, we will soon find that the reward outweighs the pain.

Jesus compares our sufferings and troubles to those of a woman in labor (John 16:20–24). The pains are hard, and they hurt! They'll make you cry, and shout, but with the hope of God's kingdom coming to earth. Pain and suffering with a purpose—pain with the deep joy of expecting prayers answered, dreams fulfilled and Christ being formed in you! Pain with the joy and excitement of a mother in labor (v. 21)—pain with the overflowing cup of God's unfathomable love, power, and blessings now and throughout eternity.

Part 1
The Cup of Kingdom
Principle
(The Prerequisite)

1

The Cup of Suffering

But Jesus answered and said, Ye know not what ye
ask. Are ye able to drink of the cup that I shall drink
of, and to be baptized with the baptism that I am
baptized with? They say unto him, We are able.
—Matthew 20:22

At the final Passover meal before His crucifixion, Jesus established one of the traditional
Jewish cups, (the third one traditionally taken after
supper), as a memorial of His death. The Lamb of
God (Jesus) instituted this cup as a symbol of His
blood that would be shed on the cross as He called
it "the new testament in my blood, which is shed for
you" (Luke 22:20).

In the Old Testament days, Jews at the Seder table
traditionally drank the third of four cups of wine called

kos b'rakhah, the cup of blessing (also called the cup of redemption). Until that point at the Passover Table, the disciples only knew that customary third cup as the cup of blessing and redemption. However, Jesus understood the Kingdom Principle and explained: in order for redemption and in order to receive the blessing, He would first have to endure the suffering, as they would also.

Earlier, Zebedee's wife had asked Jesus if her two sons (James and John) could sit with Him beside His throne in glory. Jesus responded by asking the two if they were able to drink of the cup that He would drink (Matthew 20:22). They claimed they were able to do so, to drink of the same cup, and Jesus confirmed that they indeed would.

And on that Passover evening, James and John and the other disciples drank of Jesus' bittersweet cup, including its hard-to-swallow revelation of sacrifice—as they drank, they were fellowshipping with His sufferings so they could partake of His glory. When we too, drink of His covenant cup, we're fellowshipping with His sufferings by symbolically saying, "I take this in remembrance of Your death for me and I also commit to live a life of sacrifice and self denial, and to face similar persecutions. I'll go where You go, and do what You ask me to. I pledge that I am willing to deny myself and follow You" As we make this commitment, we not only partake of His cup of suffering, but we also partake of His cup of blessing.

Later the same night, our precious Savior experienced intense agony in the Garden of Gethsemane because the time for Him to drink the whole cup of suffering. The Son of God had already tasted suffering throughout His life through much rejection and persecution, but He was about to taste death for every man. His soul became exceeding sorrowful even to the point of death (Matthew 26:38) because He was about to swallow up (defeat) death through His own sacrificial death and victorious resurrection. The pressure of the hour of the power of darkness beat Him mercilessly as He agonized in prayer; He resisted unto blood, as He strived against diabolical forces: "O my Father, if it be possible, let this cup pass from me (Matthew 26:39)." He surrendered with these words, "O my Father, if this cup may not pass away from me, except I drink it, thy will be done" (Matthew 26:42).

Jesus said He will not again drink of the fruit of the vine until He drinks it anew, with His disciples, in His Father's kingdom (Matthew 26:29). When He comes again, the cup we will drink of together won't be one of suffering, for Jesus suffered once for sin. We'll raise it together, and not only taste, but drink of it—the cup of His glory, overflowing with blessing, power, and joy.

In His humility, Jesus rode upon a donkey, but He is returning on a white horse (Revelation19:11). Because of His lowliness, He is exalted! He's bringing His trophy which is the glory cup!

And being found in fashion as a man, he humbled himself, and became obedient unto death, even the death of the cross. Wherefore God also hath highly exalted him, and given him a name which is above every name:— Philippians 2:8, 9

He's offering it to us saying "Drink from it, all of you" (Matthew 26:27b NIV). Only those who drink of His cup of suffering will drink of His cup of blessing and glory, "if so be that we suffer with him, that we may be also glorified together" (Romans 8:17b). Do you want to sup with Jesus? Just one sip and you'll say with the Psalmist:

What shall I render unto the LORD for all his benefits toward me? I will take the cup of salvation, and call upon the name of the LORD.—Psalm 116:12,13

The vessels of mercy are first seasoned with affliction, and then the wine of glory is poured in. Thus we see afflictions are beneficial to the saints.
—Thomas Watson

Prayer

Heavenly Father, I acknowledge that You are worthy of my life. Lord, I choose to take up my cross and live for You. I want to dine with You in intimate fellowship. Your Words says that You will never leave me or forsake me (Hebrews 13:5)! I praise You for demonstrating Your love for me through the sacrifice of Your Son, Jesus Christ. Amen.

2

The Cup of Reward

*Ye cannot drink the cup of the Lord, and the cup of
devils: ye cannot be partakers of the Lord's table,
and of the table of devils.*
— 1 Corinthians 10:21

Disciple of Jesus or not, you will still have to
drink a cup of suffering. But the Bible says,
"It is better, if it is God's will, to suffer for doing
good than for doing evil (1 Peter 3:17)." The cup
that the world offers may appear to be a beautiful,
enticing chalice. However, just as the Pharisees did,
the world cleans, polishes, and shines the outside of
the cup but the inside is full of greed and self-indul-
gence (Matthew 23:25 NIV). The sinful cup of the
world is the cup that Scripture reveals is in the hand
of the mother of all harlots, Mystery Babylon the

Great. "She held a golden cup in her hand, filled with abominable things and the filth of her adulteries" (Revelation 17:4b). Are you drinking of the cup of Babylon? As John the Revelator experienced when he ate the little book, the taste might be sweet in your mouth, but in your belly, it is as bitter as wormwood (Revelation 10:9). Can you think of pleasures in your life that taste sweet, but will eventually turn sour?

Moses understood the Kingdom Principle and he refused to intoxicate himself with worldly gratification:

By faith Moses, when he was come to years, refused to be called the son of Pharaoh's daughter; Choosing rather to suffer affliction with the people of God, than to enjoy the pleasures of sin for a season; Esteeming the reproach of Christ greater riches than the treasures in Egypt: for he had respect unto the recompence of the reward.

—Hebrews 11:24–26

Scripture is clear that everyone will receive a cup of reward. Those who drink the cup of suffering for the sake of Christ will also drink the cup of God's blessing! Those who drink of pleasures from the sinful cup of the world will also drink the cup of God's wrath.

For all nations have drunk of the wine of the wrath of her fornication, and the kings of the earth have committed fornication with her, and the merchants of the earth are waxed rich through the abundance of her delicacies. — Revelation 18:3

Christ has saved the best wine for last for those who gladly choose Him now and refuse to be inebriated with sinful pleasures. As Daniel refused to drink Babylon's wine, we should have that same passion for holiness (Daniel 1:8).

Oh what folly it is—for a cup of pleasure, to drink, a sea of wrath. Sin will be bitter in the end. The pleasure of sin is soon gone, but the sting remains.
—Thomas Watson

Prayer

Father, in gratitude I come before Your throne. I pray that You will give me a pure heart, so that my affections will not be set on worldly pleasures, but on You and You alone. Lord, I know that You are more than enough for me and for my every need. Your presence in my life satisfies my every desire. Lord, I surrender myself to You. Amen.

3

Fill the Cup Double

And they departed from the presence of the council,
rejoicing that they were counted worthy to suffer
shame for his name.
—Acts 5:41

Have you ever been paid time-and-a-half for working overtime? Well, double pay is even better! The reward of the righteous will be multiplied. Joseph, once despised and rejected by his brethren, received double honor when they sought him and bowed at his feet. This foreshadows the double honor that Jesus, also despised and rejected of men, will receive when the tribes of Israel bow at His feet, for it is written:

That at the name of Jesus every knee should bow, of things in heaven, and things in earth, and things under the earth; And that every tongue should confess that Jesus Christ is Lord, to the glory of God the Father.

—Philippians 2:10, 11

Double pay, however, is to be feared by the unrighteous, for God will repay the unrepentant double for their evil deeds:

Reward her even as she rewarded you, and double unto her double according to her works: in the cup which she hath filled fill to her double....Therefore shall her plagues come in one day, death, and mourning, and famine; and she shall be utterly burned with fire: for strong is the Lord God who judgeth her—Revelation 18:6, 8

Jesus warned that if men persecuted Him, they would likewise persecute His disciples and if they believed His sayings, they would believe ours. Just as He is recompensed in this end-time hour, His disciples who are faithfully serving Him will be recompensed as well.

Hear the word of the LORD, ye that tremble at his word; your brethren that hated you, that cast you out for my name's sake, said, Let the LORD be glorified: but he shall appear to your joy, and they shall be ashamed.—Isaiah 66:5

This is why Jesus calls us blessed when persecuted:

Blessed are ye, when men shall revile you, and persecute you, and shall say all manner of evil against you falsely, for my sake. Rejoice, and be exceeding glad: for great is your reward in heaven: for so persecuted they the prophets which were before you.—Matthew 5:11, 12

It's truly a privilege to suffer for the cause of Christ. The apostles were beaten, and rejoiced that they were counted worthy to suffer shame for His name (Acts 5:41)! In the book of Hebrews we read of many Old Testament saints who suffered severely for the sake of the Word of God, those "(Of whom the world was not worthy:)" (Hebrews 11:38a). Scripture also says that they did not receive the promise. "God having provided some better thing for us, that they without us should not be made perfect." (Hebrews 11:40). For they suffered before Christ came to the earth, but we who suffer for the sake of the Great Commission fill up that which is behind of the afflictions of Christ for his body's sake, which is the church (Colossians 1:24).

There are no crown-wearers in heaven who were not cross bearers here below.
—Charles Haddon Spurgeon

Prayer

Father, Your Word says that every knee shall bow and every tongue confess that Jesus Christ is Lord to the glory of God of the Father (Philippians 2:10,11). Lord, I choose to serve You now. Thank You for Your presence that dwells in me. Amen.

Part 2
It's Not Strange to Suffer

4

For Christ's Sake

*Beloved, think it not strange concerning the fiery
trial which is to try you, as though some strange
thing happened unto you: But rejoice, inasmuch as
ye are partakers of Christ's sufferings; that, when
his glory shall be revealed, ye may be
glad also with exceeding joy.*
—1 Peter 4:12, 13

The Bible speaks of many strange things
including strange gods, strange women, strange
fire and incense, and even strange waters. But one
thing it tells us not to think strange is our suffering
for Christ's sake.

Saints have suffered throughout all of the ages.
If we think that once we become Christians we
won't have to suffer, we will soon discover quite the

contrary. The difference is that our suffering now has purpose. Instead of suffering for our sin, we suffer for righteousness. Instead of suffering being strange for Christians, it's necessary, mandatory, and required. It's strange to indulge in lusts and serve false gods. It's strange to live life as an experience, having no God-given purpose, but relying on limited human efforts, chance and luck. The biblical strangers were the "-ites"— the Canaanites, Jebusites and others who did not have a covenant relationship with the God of Israel. But for favor-ites (those walking with God whom have found favor in His sight) it never has been strange to suffer. Christ said, "The disciple is not above his master, nor the servant above his lord" (Matthew 10:24). Therefore, if Christ suffered, then we should expect to suffer. "For unto you it is given in the behalf of Christ, not only to believe on him, but also to suffer for his sake;" (Philippians 1:29).

When we suffer for our faith, we should remain faithful with our hearts fixed on the salvation of God. Though the pain can be beyond words and almost unbearable at times, it is always worth it to continue in trust and obedience because there is a greater future glory. If we rejoice in suffering for the sake of Jesus, then we will share in His glory. We'll rejoice now but be overjoyed then.

There won't be any suffering in heaven. Our suffering is only for a season. But it's worth it. It's pain with a purpose—a greater purpose than we can ever imagine.

Don't look forward to the day you stop suffering,
because when it comes you'll know you're dead.
—Tennessee Williams, London Observer (1958)

Prayer

Father, I don't want to be a stranger to Your presence. Fill me with Your Holy Spirit that I may dwell in covenant with You through Your Son. Open the eyes of my heart's understanding—I want to know You, Lord.

5

It is Written

And said unto them, Thus it is written, and thus it
behoved Christ to suffer, and to rise from
the dead the third day:
—Luke 24:46

Behooved means it was necessary (as binding).
If it was necessary for Christ to suffer, then it
certainly is for His followers. As much as we don't
want to suffer, it is often necessary for God's glory
as well as our benefit—that is why "It is written."
As Christians we often declare "It is written" in
spiritual combat, following the example of Christ in
the wilderness. But we need to remember that Jesus
referred to what "is written" in regard to His suffering
as well. When He was in the Garden of Gethsemane,
He emphatically implied that He could easily beckon

twelve legions of angels to deliver Him, through prayer to the Father, and the reason He resisted doing so was that He knew what was written. He said, "But how then would the Scriptures be fulfilled that say it must happen in this way?" (Matthew 26:54 NIV).

Jesus knew what was written, and that it was destined to come to pass; this gave Him the steadfastness and readiness to endure until the end. His foreknowledge prepared Him for the battle. In order to prepare us for the battle, He has forewarned us. He said, "In the world ye shall have tribulation:" (John 16:33b). Jesus prepared us for trials and persecutions that we face in the world. He said, "But these things have I told you, that when the time shall come, ye may remember that I told you of them. And these things I said not unto you at the beginning, because I was with you" (John 16:4). There is such comfort in knowing that our sufferings for Christ's sake are not in vain, but God has allowed them for a reason. They will ultimately work together for our good and His glory. There is great security in knowing that God is sovereign and our lives are in His hands. Since we know it is written and the Lord has already warned us of things to come, we can be ready, endure, and stand strong.

God promises deliverance in trouble — He doesn't promise deliverance from trouble. But He assures us and tells us to be of good cheer, because He has overcome the world, and there is nothing for us to fear. We don't have to think that it is strange to suffer because it's not strange; it is written!

No pain, no palm, no thorns, no throne, no gall, no glory, no cross, no crown.
—William Penn, No Cross, No Crown

Prayer

Father, endow me with supernatural strength and prepare me for the high calling. Thank You Lord that greater is Jesus Christ that is in me than the enemy that is in the world (1 John 4:4). Empower me with Your presence and let my life be spent on Your purposes.

6

Armed and Dangerous:
Revelation—A Mighty Weapon

Forasmuch then as Christ hath suffered for us in the flesh, arm yourselves likewise with the same mind: for he that hath suffered in the flesh hath ceased from sin;
—1 Peter 4:1

When we, as believers, come to the revelation that nothing Satan can do to us is against us, but rather it is working for us, we become armed with a mighty weapon against him. Satan could not succeed in his temptation of Jesus in the wilderness, because Jesus knew what He was called to do. Isaiah prophesied that by Jesus' knowledge He would justify many (53:11). Jesus knew that He was called to suffer, and that is why He asked His disciples, "the cup which my Father hath given me, shall I not drink it?" (John 18:11). Armed with this revelation knowledge, He was willing to suffer. Jesus didn't want to suffer, but He was willing. He said, "nevertheless not my will, but thine, be done" (Luke 22:42b).

When we are mentally prepared to suffer, we will not fear man, harm, isolation, and other afflictions. If we will bear the mindset that Christ demonstrated while on earth, then, we will not be like the children of Israel who murmured because of their lack of food and water. Rather, we will be like Paul who did not speak in respect of want, but learned in whatsoever state to be content. Paul knew both how to be abased and how to abound. Everywhere and in all things, he knew how to be full and to be hungry, both to abound and to suffer need. Paul could do all things through Christ who strengthened him (Philippians 4:13). We should all, like Paul, have the mindset of Jesus Christ, who though He was reviled, reviled not again (1 Peter 2:23). "He was oppressed, and he was afflicted, yet he opened not his mouth:" (Isaiah 53:7).

Jesus rebuked the disciples on the road to Emmaus for not believing what is written, as spoken by the prophets. (This reveals that the prophets foretold of Christ's suffering and glorification.) He called them fools and slow of heart (Luke 24:25). A fool is someone who doesn't believe God, and that is why He rebuked them for being "slow of heart to believe all that the prophets have spoken. Ought not Christ to have suffered these things, and to enter into his glory?" (Luke 24:25, 26). We too should know that in order to enter into His glory; we have to suffer with Him. Since it is written for Christ to suffer, it follows that His disciples will suffer too. Why is it written that Christ and His followers must suffer? The Bible says that Christ learned obedience through the things that He suffered (Hebrews 5:8). Don't we learn as well? Suffering can teach us great lessons and accomplish great things in us.

If the disciples had believed the prophets, they wouldn't have been so sad. Rather they leaned on their own understanding and were despondent about His death saying, "but we had hoped that he was the one who was going to redeem Israel." (Luke 24:21a NIV). They were shortsighted and did not apply God's victorious Word. They did not know that Christ's suffering was for something far beyond and better, therefore Jesus rebuked them. The Bible admonishes us, as well, to believe God. To avoid being foolish, we need to focus on the victory found in God's Word and rejoice at trials and tribulations, knowing that they are working for our good and that our pain is our gain.

And he said unto them, These are the words which I spake unto you, while I was yet with you, that all things must be fulfilled, which were written in the law of Moses, and in the prophets, and in the psalms, concerning me. Then opened he their understanding, that they might understand the scriptures.

—Luke 24:44, 45.

The prophets therefore, foretold of Christ's sufferings, and the salvation, grace, and glory in trial and tribulation. Later, Peter wrote of the glory of Christ and His followers through his epistles, namely:

Beloved, think it not strange concerning the fiery trial which is to try you, as though some strange thing happened unto you: But rejoice, inasmuch as ye are partakers of Christ's sufferings; that, when his glory shall be revealed, ye may be glad also with exceeding joy. If ye be reproached for the name of Christ, happy are ye; for the spirit of glory and of God resteth upon you...Yet if any man suffer as a Christian, let him not be ashamed; but let him glorify God on this behalf.— 1 Peter 4:12–16

This "glory" is not only revealed at Christ's coming but now in our suffering, the suffering of Christians up to and in this present age. This doesn't preclude the glory to come, but it is glory to glory.

Pray and ask God to open your spiritual eyes and understanding to the work of the cross and of His overwhelming love. Ask Him to open up your heart, and quicken it, to believe Him in all things.

If we suffer, we will also reign with him.
—2 Timothy 2:12a

Prayer

Father, I acknowledge that only when I seek You can I gain the revelation that will help me to stand firm in my faith. Only when I seek You can I find peace that surpasses all understanding. Lord, I pray for a passion to seek You; a passion to know You and Your will for my life. Lord, I want to see You now more than ever—let Your power overtake me. I surrender all. In Jesus' name. Amen.

7

Worthy

*Which is a manifest token of the righteous judg-
ment of God, that ye may be counted worthy of the
kingdom of God, for which ye also suffer:*
—2 Thessalonians 1:5

Your pain has worth. Suffering relates to worthi-
ness in the kingdom of God (2 Thessalonians
1:5). This does not mean that God takes pleasure in
suffering. Rather, Satan is the one who takes pleasure
in your pain, and he certainly doesn't want it to be for
your gain. Satan wants to wreak havoc in your life
causing you to suffer in vain, without expanding the
kingdom of God. In Matthew 17:15 we read about a
boy sorely vexed by evil spirits. The root meaning of
sore is "worthless," and vexed refers to "suffering."
This boy was grievously and worthlessly suffering

because of evil spirits. It's better to suffer for God than to suffer for the devil.

The apostles rejoiced that they were counted worthy to suffer shame for His name (Acts 5:41). They gladly risked their lives for the name of our Lord Jesus Christ. The Lamb of God is worthy to receive glory, honor, and praise from mankind because He was slain on our behalf. His death made him worthy to take the book and open the seals (Revelation 5:9). Through death to sin and a life of obedience in Christ, we can become worthy of eternal rewards. When God calls us unto Himself it's because of His grace, not because we are worthy. But those who are given much and receive rewards from God do so because they are worthy of it (Revelation 3:4). A reward is something offered for service or achievement. Those who are faithful with little, God will trust with much (Luke 19:17). As the saying goes, "No pain, no gain!" If we suffer for Christ, we will be counted worthy to reign with Christ (2 Timothy 2:12). Jesus said, "And he that taketh not his cross, and followeth after me, is not worthy of me. He that findeth his life shall lose it: and he that loseth his life for my sake shall find it (Matthew 10:38, 39). All the riches and treasures of Egypt were not of any worth compared with the worth of the pain Moses would face for God. Therefore, Moses esteemed the reproach of Christ. He thought highly of it and exalted it. Moses appreciated the pain because he knew it was to his gain; "for he had respect unto the recompence of the reward" (Hebrews 11:26b).

Understanding why God, at times, allows you to face difficult situations helps fortify your faith so that you will not be shaken in the fierce storms of life. Realize that there can be positive qualities etched into your character due to the cellar of suffering. Some of the qualities are bravery, courage, patience, steadfastness, perseverance, humility, self-control, boldness, a peaceful heart, a tender heart, greater empathy, greater compassion, increased faith and trust in the Lord. So too, suffering can plow the heart to erase many bad characteristics, such as: pride, self-centeredness, arrogance, hard heartedness, critical or judgmental attitudes, narcissism, religiosity, bad tempers, and abusiveness.

Looking back, I clearly see
All the grief that had to be
Left me when the pain was o'er
Richer than I'd been before.
—Anonymous

Prayer

Lord, I believe that You are purging me and refining me and though I pass through the fire, I will not be burned, but will come forth as pure gold. Give me strength, Father, to endure and to be unmovable. I declare, Your Word, that no weapon formed against me can prosper (Isaiah 54:17) and if God is with me who can be against me (Romans 8:31)? You are my life and the One I seek to please.

8

Appointed to Suffer

For I will shew him how great things he must suffer
for my name's sake.
—Acts 9:16

Like Christ, Christians are appointed to suffer. The Apostle Paul, previous to his conversion, ensured that Christians would suffer for their faith. During Paul's conversion experience, the Lord told Ananias that He would show Paul how great things he must suffer for His name's sake (Acts 9:16). Though some have suggested Paul's suffering as a type of punishment for his persecution of Christians, it was the high call of God on his life that required him to suffer, in order for him to share in Christ's glory. In Second Corinthians we find that God allowed Paul to suffer, lest Paul should exalt himself above measure for the divine revelations from the Lord (12:7). We can see how suffering was an integral part of Paul's call, because Paul described in the New Testament how his sufferings resulted in the advancement of the Gospel of the Lord Jesus Christ.

As all believers, Paul was called to reflect the character of the Lord Jesus Christ, and he acknowledged that sufferings allowed the transformation to take place. Therefore, Paul rejoiced in his sufferings and counted them a privilege, acknowledging that without the call of God on his life he wouldn't have been shipwrecked three times, beaten, stoned and more. But neither would he be rewarded with crowns, glory, and eternal life. Paul should serve as a genuine example of Christians who don't want to lose part in the eternal weight of glory. Like Paul, we shouldn't be so quick to want to escape sufferings. It may very well be a principle that the greater the call, the greater the suffering.

Like Paul, you can acknowledge that the right perspective and positive attitude can take a lot of pain out of the thorn that's in your side; for His grace is sufficient for you. "And we know that all things work together for good to them that love God, to them who are the called according to his purpose" (Romans 8:28).

Paul didn't escape suffering until he left his earthly tabernacle. It is believed that he was beheaded under Nero's reign. Paul wrote of death in the book of Philippians and said that he had a desire to depart because he knew it was far better to be with Christ (1:23).

Paul wasn't the only apostle who suffered intensely. As we recall the history of the apostles, we find that most or all of them experienced brutal deaths during persecutions. Some were beheaded, crucified, stabbed, and beaten. And multitudes of other devout Christians throughout history have suffered horrible deaths through horrendous acts of persecution. Although its sobering, it is also assuring to know that faithful followers of Christ embraced the martyrs' deaths, choosing a better resurrection.

According to <u>Foxe's Christian Martyrs of the World</u>, written by John Foxe:

- Stephen: The Jews gnashed their teeth at him and stoned him.
- James the brother of John: Beheaded in AD 36.
- Thomas: Martyred in India.
- Simon, brother of Jude and James the younger: Crucified in Egypt during the reign of Emperor Trajan.
- Simon the Zealot: Crucified.
- Mark: Burned to death.
- Bartholomew: Beaten, crucified, and beheaded in Armenia.
- Andrew, Peter's brother: Crucified by a governor named Aegeas. As he approached the place of crucifixion, he said, "O cross, most welcome and longed for! With a willing mind, joyfully and desirously, I come to you, being the scholar of Him which did hang on you, because I have

always been your lover and yearned to embrace you."

- Matthew: Killed with a spear by someone sent by King Hircanus.
- Philip: Stoned and crucified.
- James: Thrown off the temple and killed when someone him in the head.
- Peter: Crucified upside-down.

Though we may not face such violent sufferings as did these brave souls, suffering is still a key part of our Christian walk. We don't usually view suffering and trials as highlights of our Christian walk. But what indeed should be our view toward suffering? What role does it play in our lives?

We can experience and endure sufferings because Christ first suffered for us. The power and the glory of God were revealed through Christ's sufferings. It's because of obedience and love that we too must suffer. In fact, we are called to suffer, and to endure it patiently. This is my calling, and this is your calling. This is the calling of every believer in Christ.

but if, when ye do well, and suffer for it, ye take it patiently, this is acceptable with God. For even hereunto were ye called: because Christ also suffered for us, leaving us an example, that ye should follow his steps:
— 1 Peter 2:20b, 21

The Word of God reveals to us the wonderful effects suffering can have on lives submitted to the Lord; including ceasing from sin, (1 Peter 4:1), learning obedience (Hebrews 5:8), and being made strong, firm and steadfast (1 Peter 5:10 NIV).

Afflictions add to the saints' glory. The more the diamond is cut, the more it sparkles, the heavier the saints cross, the heavier will be their crown.
—Thomas Watson

Prayer

Lord, take my heart and form it; my life and transform it and my will and conform it to Yours. Give me Your joy O' Lord, even in the face of persecution, knowing that what the enemy means for evil, You turn it to my good and Your glory. Thank You, Lord! Amen.

9

In the Midst of Joy

*Many a time have they afflicted me from my youth,
may Israel now say: Many a time have they afflicted
me from my youth: yet they have not prevailed
against me.*
—Psalm 129:1,2

Israel has suffered so many afflictions that the Jews identify with and take claim to the Old Testament prophecies of the Messiah's sufferings. The same Scriptures that speak of Christ also relate to the sufferings of Israel. As the chosen people of God, they have endured much tribulation. This applies both to the natural and to the spiritual.

Jewish weddings are celebrated with great expressions of joy, filled with laughter, dancing, feasting and more. However, in the midst of the joyous occasion there remains a sobering tradition that may be the best-known element of all the wedding symbols. At the height of personal joy, sadness is recalled by the shattering of a glass. A prevalent interpretation is that the breaking of glass serves as a reminder of the destruction of the Temple in Jerusalem.

For some, the interpretation is broadened to represent all the losses suffered by the Jewish people. Although the wedding provides a taste of redemption, the sorrow of a broken world remains. Likewise every year, as Jews celebrate the great deliverance from the bondage of slavery in Egypt at the Passover feast, they partake of the bitter herbs as a reminder of their suffering.

The Jews have been long acquainted with suffering. Likewise, Christians have an underlying sorrow even in the midst of joy. The joy of the Lord is our strength, yet in a fallen world there is a sound of brokenness reverberating in our spirits. We may be more cognizant of the world's decadence since we are eagerly anticipating the restoration, but all creation is subject to its despair and is longing for redemption.

For we know that the whole creation groaneth and travaileth in pain together until now. And not only they, but ourselves also, which have the firstfruits of the Spirit, even we ourselves groan within ourselves, waiting for the adoption, to wit, the redemption of our body. — Romans 8:22, 23

Though paradoxical, Scripture shows that things meant to scatter often gather. For example, the persecution of the early church at Jerusalem scattered the believers abroad, but their scattering resulted in gathering more people into the kingdom of God as believers went out preaching the Word (Acts 11:21).

Suffering is actually what brings the restoration of all things. We can see this in the sufferings of John the Baptist, who came with the spirit of Elijah to restore all things.

And he answered and told them, Elias verily cometh first, and restoreth all things; and how it is written of the Son of man, that he must suffer many things, and be set at nought. — Mark 9:12

And of course, we also see the epitome of this principle in the life of Jesus, who came as a suffering servant to fulfill the law. The One who suffered the most is the One who brings the most relief of suffering — redemption to a fallen world.

I cry because I'm joyful and I cry because I'm sad. Let my every cry hasten the Lord's return and His kingdom which will dry every tear.

—Yapheh PhiYah

Prayer

Lord, put my tears into Your bottle (Psalm 56:8). I believe that You are going to pour out Your power in response to my heart's cry. Hearken O'Lord to my prayers; hear the voice of my supplication and come quickly.

Part 3
Dying to Live

10

The Tearing Away

*Therefore also now, saith the LORD, turn ye even to
me with all your heart, and with fasting, and with
weeping, and with mourning:*
—Joel 2:12

Dedicating your life to the Lord, means change
and change often includes suffering. Being
delivered from the dysfunctional lifestyle of compro-
mise, complacency, and status quo sometimes
involves some serious pain. We have to tear ourselves
away from worldly attachments, or have them ripped
away from us in order for our lives to be redefined.
This can include our own theories, bias opinions, and
self-made policies. It often also includes unhealthy
relationships and selfish priorities.

Sanctification is the process of being made holy, but the word means "the act of being set apart." This holy seclusion requires an abandonment of worldly lusts and denial of fleshly indulgences. God insists that His people be holy, for without holiness no man can see God (Hebrews 12:14). Praise God, through Jesus, our sanctification is progressive. We are sanctified, being sanctified, and will be sanctified. Of course, this also means we are set apart, being set apart, and will be set apart for His glory.

As we discover our true identity in Christ, our worldly support systems begin to crumble, including our pride, policies, and success systems. We realize that who we are does not merely depend on our physical appearance, income, or the acceptance and judgments of others. We have to rid ourselves of the pride that seeks to conform to the standards of society, and realign our standards to God's mandates.

But isn't it better for you to rend your heart from ungodliness, than to allow Satan to rend you sore as he seeks to destroy your life with false support systems, and relationships that are not built on a biblical foundation (John 10:10)? Crisis can separate us from those things that aren't essential for our destinies and callings. But then the question remains, "If we wouldn't have held on to them so tightly, would we have to go through certain crises?" We can not always control every situation and circumstance, but there are some we can; especially as we align our hearts with the Word of God and trade our selfishness for a deep, intimate relationship with the Lord.

The tearing of your heart unto repentance can include holy tears, but Satan's tearing of souls produces tears of torment. The reality of the spiritual battle and the diabolical works of the enemy are evident in the Bible. A deaf and dumb spirit gripped a little boy and tore him, causing him to gnash his teeth and pine away (Mark 9:18). This was an extreme case of possession, but reveals Satan's intention to tear up lives and souls. David prayed to the Lord for deliverance from his persecutor "Lest he tear my soul like a lion, rending it in pieces, while there is none to deliver" (Psalm 7:2).

Through prayer and intercession, we can liberate ourselves from familiar spirits and soul ties. As we tear our hearts in contrition and cleave to the Lord, our lives will sever from the love of worldliness. "Love not the world, neither the things that are in the world. If any man love the world, the love of the Father is not in him" (1 John 2:15). We become new through the righteousness of Christ, believing God's promises and plans for our lives. Oh, what relief it brings us to endure the incisions of spiritual surgery for holiness' sake, rather than to be slaughtered by Satan's rage and God's judgment. "Now consider this, ye that forget God, lest I tear you in pieces, and there be none to deliver" (Psalm 50:22).

The calling of the Christian is an enlistment for one's entire being and a mandate to detach oneself from many in order to be attached to One.
—Unknown

Prayer

Lord, I surrender to You the things of the world—those things that I cleave to that keep me from drawing close to You. Take it all, Lord. Set me free from the bondages of deception. I surrender all of my worldly plans, goals, desires, and dreams; because You hold my destiny in Your hands. I want to live for You. I give You my life. In Jesus' name. Amen.

11

Stripped to be Decked

For where your treasure is, there will your heart be also.
—Matthew 6:21

Where is your treasure? What are you truly cherishing? It will reveal your true love. In today's society, it's difficult to relinquish love for material things. It's easy to become focused on worldly possessions since we live in the midst of such commercialism. Jesus said that we cannot serve God and mammon (the false god of riches and avarice) (Matthew 6:24).

God requires His people to be stripped of the worldly mindset. The Lord does not desire us to suffer the curse of poverty, but He desires a pure heart that's fixed on Him above all else. He doesn't want us to regard temporal wealth more than His presence, but rather to store up heavenly treasures by making our primary focus in life on living for Him. Jesus said, "And again I say unto you, It is easier for a camel to go through the eye of a needle, than for a rich man to enter into the kingdom of God." (Matthew 19:24). Some claim that the "eye of the needle" was a narrow gate in Jerusalem that travelers on camels could pass through only by stripping off the loads of goods. The disciples in response asked Jesus, "Who then can be saved?" And Jesus told them that with God all things are possible (Matthew 19:25b, 26).

Our love for God will compel us to rid ourselves of worldly attachments that hinder our relationship with Him. Jesus told the rich man to go sell all his goods and give alms, and he would have treasure in heaven (Matthew 19:21). But because he refused to suffer the loss of temporal possessions in order to gain spiritually, he went away sorrowful. Those who insist on cherishing worldly things more than kingdom possessions will likewise end up very sorrowful.

When we suffer for a season to be stripped of our lusts, we will be recompensed with a storehouse of blessings. If we suffer to lose our sinful lusts, we will gain much more through our love for God. Moses considered the reproach of Christ greater riches than the treasures of Egypt and soon discovered that God is the One who gives power to get wealth that He may establish His covenant (Deuteronomy 8:17). Moses learned about God's good treasure for those who keep His commandments.

The LORD shall open unto thee his good treasure, the heaven to give the rain unto thy land in his season, and to bless all the work of thine hand: and thou shalt lend unto many nations, and thou shalt not borrow
— Deuteronomy 28:12

God will bless us abundantly when our hearts and minds are set on Him. God has a treasure for everyone, and will reveal it in due season. Some are treasuring up His blessings and others, His wrath.

If we strip away our lusts, we'll be decked with glory. Because Jesus stripped Himself of His heavenly glory and humbled Himself to become a man, He is now adorned with many crowns (Revelation 19:12). If we share in Christ's sufferings through loss for His name's sake, we will also share in His glory (Romans 8:17). Glory can be defined as wealth in both the physical and spiritual realms. Jesus told a parable about the kingdom of heaven. He said that the kingdom is like a treasure hidden in a field. When a man finds it, he goes and sells everything he owns and buys the field (Matthew 13:44). As you sacrifice for Christ's sake, you gain the treasure of the kingdom now and through out eternity.

And Jesus answered and said, Verily I say unto you, There is no man that hath left house, or brethren, or sisters, or father, or mother, or wife, or children, or lands, for my sake, and the gospel's, But he shall receive an hundredfold now in this time, houses, and brethren, and sisters, and mothers, and children, and lands, with persecutions; and in the world to come eternal life. — Mark 10:29, 30

Whether you are reaping the hundredfold return now or not, you can be certain of recompense for everything you willingly offer. In the book of Revelation, Jesus said to the church of Smyrna, "I know your afflictions and your poverty—yet you are rich" (Revelation 2:9a NIV). If our hearts are right with God, then we can rejoice in our suffering, because our pain is wealth. That is why Paul took pleasure in neediness, because it strengthened his reliance upon God (2 Corinthians 12:10). It was in a time of famine that God put treasures in the sacks of Israel's children (Genesis 43:23). The more we rely upon God, the more we find that He provides all our needs according to His riches and glory (Philippians 4:19).

About us are a thousand 'entangling' things. This world is very much like the pools we have heard of in India, in which grows a long grass of so clinging a character that, if a man once falls into the water, it is almost certain to be his death, for only with the utmost difficulty could he be rescued from the meshes of the deadly, weedy net, which immediately wraps itself around him. This world is even thus entangling. All the efforts of grace are needed to preserve men from being ensnared with the deceitfulness of riches and the cares of this life.
—Charles Haddon Spurgeon

Prayer

God of Wonders beyond our universe and galaxy—You are beautiful beyond description, too marvelous for words. Keep my eyes focused on You, Father, above all else. Let every thing I am and everything I have be for Your glory. Thank You for every thing You have blessed me with, Lord, for I know that every good and perfect gift comes from heaven above (James 1:17). Amen.

12

The Spoiling of the Goods

For ye had compassion of me in my bonds, and took joyfully the spoiling of your goods, knowing in yourselves that ye have in heaven a better and an enduring substance.
—Hebrews 10:34

Are you ready to spoil yourself? Before you answer, let's look at the definition of "spoiling" in the biblical sense. In order to understand the meaning, think of spoiling in terms of "spoiling" the enemy. Plundering the enemy's camp or taking all the enemy's goods is seen often in the Old Testament. Now we see this same term in the New Testament, not referring to Christians who spoiled the enemy, but to Christians who spoiled THEMSELVES. That's right, they allowed their goods to be taken in order to support and further the Gospel of Jesus Christ. The Bible says that those who gave so graciously have in heaven a better and enduring substance (Hebrews 10:34).

You've heard it said that you can't out-give God. That's because He graciously gives above and beyond what we could ever sacrifice to Him. In the book of Philippians, we read how Paul addressed those who met his monetary needs through free-will offerings. He claimed that it was fruit to their account and furthermore described it as an odor of sweet smell, a sacrifice acceptable, well pleasing to God (4:18). Isn't this true of all of our free-will offerings to the Lord; whether it be our money, our time, our prayers, our tears? God promises that what we dedicate, surrender, and commit to Him yields eternal dividends. The gifts the Church gave profited the spread of the Gospel in their day, advanced the kingdom, put a blessing on their lives, and stored up heavenly rewards throughout eternity. No wonder we should spoil ourselves for the sake of the Lord. When we give to the Lord, we stand upon His promises, which bring great joy because they are eternal treasures. David said, "I rejoice at thy word, as one that findeth great spoil" (Psalm119:162). So, it is those who spoil themselves, for Christ's sake, who actually end up with all the goods.

Saints gain more by their losses than by their profits.
—Charles Haddon Spurgeon

Prayer

Father, I come before You, surrendering my life to You completely. Thank You for the power and authority of Your Word. Help me to keep my heart and mind fixed and stayed upon You. Help me to remain steadfast, unmovable, always abounding in the work of the Lord (1 Corinthians 15:58). In Jesus' name. Amen.

13

Shedding the Shell of Carnality

For if ye live after the flesh, ye shall die: but if ye through the Spirit do mortify the deeds of the body, ye shall live.
—Romans 8:13

God's love was revealed perfectly through Christ's suffering. The ultimate victory over death and hell was accomplished through Jesus' death on the cross and His resurrection! Through death came forth life and life more abundantly! This is a principle of creation. For example, a seed planted in the ground has to die and lose its shell in order to spring up life. This is why it is such a privilege to suffer for the sake of Christ. As we die to our sinful nature and lose the shell of our carnality, our spirits can be quickened with the resurrection power of God.

Only when we die to our selfish ways and our carnal lusts can we walk in the Spirit of God. Jesus said, "He that loveth his life shall lose it; and he that hateth his life in this world shall keep it unto life eternal" (John 12:25). The Bible says the flesh and the spirit are at enmity with one another. "For to be carnally minded is death; but to be spiritually minded is life and peace" (Romans 8:6). Self-denial or abstinence from worldly pleasures is suffering for the sake of Christ. Again, it is much better to suffer for Christ than to suffer for seasonal pleasures of sin. "For the wages of sin is death" (Romans 6:23a).

As Jesus denied Himself and was crucified on the cross, we are called to deny ourselves and crucify the flesh with its affections and lusts. "For he that is dead is freed from sin" (Romans 6:7). Self-denial is not a common concept in this age of self indulgence. Nevertheless, it is the essence of our Christian walk. Each believer in Christ is a new creation (2 Corinthians 5:17 NIV). The more we deny ourselves, the more our carnal tendencies pass away and we can be transformed by the renewing of our minds. For the sake of Christ, we are to deny our own agendas, ambitions, goals, and dreams that are not in line with God's will for our lives. Likewise, we are to deny materialistic idols, habits, ungodly relationships and everything else that hinders our relationship with the Lord.

Jesus said that no one who puts his hand to the plow and looks back is fit for the kingdom of God (Luke 9:62). We are to reckon ourselves dead to sin and to our past sinful lifestyles and alive unto God through Jesus Christ our Lord (Romans 6:11). Paul wrote in the book of Philippians, "but this one thing I do, forgetting those things which are behind, and reaching forth unto those things which are before, I press toward the mark for the prize of the high calling of God in Christ Jesus" (Philippians 3:13b, 14). Of course, as we forsake past times, we find that persecutions always follow. "Yea, and all that will live godly in Christ Jesus shall suffer persecution" (2 Timothy 3:12). This is especially evident as we seek to fulfill the Great Commission; reaching souls for Christ. There are many who refuse to hear the Word of God and rage against those who spread the Gospel. We can find consolation in the words of the Messiah who told us in advance of the enmities we would face. Jesus warned us that we, being His servants, would face opposition too. Jesus' persecution fulfilled His destiny to die, which in turn enabled Him to rise from the dead. Likewise, through persecution, we have fellowship with Christ's sufferings and partake of His resurrection power. Like gold which is refined in the fire, we pass through the fires of persecution. As we are tried and tested, we are conformed unto His death. In Second Corinthians, Paul spoke of the manifestation of Christ's life through persecutions and afflictions:

We are troubled on every side, yet not distressed; we are perplexed, but not in despair; Persecuted, but not forsaken; cast down, but not destroyed; Always bearing about in the body the dying of the Lord Jesus, that the life also of Jesus might be made manifest in our body. — 2 Corinthians 4:8–10

Suffering for Christ is a small price to pay to live and receive an eternal weight of glory. Praise God! This promise applies both to this life and to the life to come! The more we abstain from carnal desires, and seek eternal values, the more the power of God is revealed in us. Moreover, as we are persecuted for His sake, we inherit the kingdom of heaven, and as we are conformed to His death and partake of His resurrection, the greater the anointing manifest on our lives.

As it is written, For thy sake we are killed all the day long; we are accounted as sheep for the slaughter. Nay, in all these things we are more than conquerors through him that loved us. — Romans 8:36,37

Rather than death conquering us, we are conquering through our death to self because only when we get out of the way can Christ-likeness manifest. Instead of listening to our own formulated opinions, we submit to the Word of God and the voice of the Holy Spirit. Instead of relying on our arbitrary emotions, we stand in faith believing what God's Word says and instead of conforming to the depraved standards of our degenerate society; we seek to please the Father. As we are transformed by the renewing of our minds, we are "more than conquerors" through Christ. A conqueror is one who overcomes. It's through our death to self that we are changed through the victorious life of Christ. Thus, the more we are transformed into the image of Christ, the more fruit we bear. "But the fruit of the Spirit is love, joy, peace, longsuffering, gentleness, goodness, faith" (Galatians 5:22). Life is all the more pleasant when we abide in the Vine and bring forth fruit! And not only do we enjoy this life in the presence of God, but also His glory shall be revealed in us beyond measure throughout eternity!

To be despised, to be spit upon, and to be carica-
tured, and to be jeered, is the highest honor that a
Christian can have.
—Charles Haddon Spurgeon

Prayer

Heavenly Father, victory belongs to You. Thank You for sending Your Son to defeat death, hell and the grave. Let the resurrection power of Christ Jesus reign in me as I deny myself and surrender my life into Your hands. Lord, change and transform me into Your likeness. Change this heart inside of me. In Jesus' mighty name, Amen.

Part 4
Choosing Life

14

The Land of the Righteous:
A Lily Among Thorns

*Instead of the thorn shall come up the fir tree, and
instead of the brier shall come up the myrtle tree:
and it shall be to the LORD for a name, for an everlasting sign that shall not be cut off.*
—Isaiah 55:13

Thorns are the fruit of a fallen world and we all
at times have felt their pricking pain. Because
we've experienced the fruit of the fall, or the pain
and suffering that this world offers; we can now
know and grasp the beauty of salvation.

God allows this pain and uses it to push us
towards change and revival. Through it, He creates
in us, the excellence of His glory. The crown of

thorns that pierced Jesus' brow enabled Him to wear many crowns (Revelation 19:12) and likewise, certain thorns can enable God's children to receive the crown of life (James 1:12). Just as thorns are a significant part of the growth of beautiful roses, they are conducive to the maturity of the Body of Christ. In the Song of Solomon, the beloved is described, "As the lily among thorns" (2:2).

Consider the Apostle Paul. He wrestled with a trial so sharp he called it a "thorn in the flesh". Nevertheless, God not only told Paul that His grace was sufficient for him, but that His strength is made perfect in weakness (2 Corinthians 12:9). God's strength manifests in our weakness, frailty, and suffering. Consequently, it's through frailty and brokenness that God best uses us.

God allows us to be broken, but through Jesus Christ, we are made whole. Our peace doesn't come from the world, but from Christ. This is a peace that transcends any peace this world may offer. Jesus said, "Peace I leave with you, my peace I give unto you: not as the world giveth, give I unto you. Let not your heart be troubled, neither let it be afraid" (John 14:27).

Paul said that we are to learn to be content in any situation. He knew he was in God's will, regardless of the circumstances, regardless of what he had to endure. He wrote,

Who shall separate us from the love of Christ? shall tribulation, or distress, or persecution, or famine, or nakedness, or peril, or sword? As it is written, For thy sake we are killed all the day long; we are accounted as sheep for the slaughter. Nay, in all these things we are more than conquerors through him that loved us. For I am persuaded, that neither death, nor life, nor angels, nor principalities, nor powers, nor things present, nor things to come, Nor height, nor depth, nor any other creature, shall be able to separate us from the love of God, which is in Christ Jesus our Lord. — Romans 8:35–39

Jesus did not pray that the Father would take His disciples out of the world, but He did pray for the Father's protection from evil (John 17:15). Such evil is like poisonous thorns. If the Israelites didn't drive out the wicked nations, those nations would become thorns in their sides that would vex them. Likewise, we are not to allow the thorns of sin to choke us. If we do not take heed to the ways of God, we can bring pain upon ourselves and others. Briers and thorns are symbolic of the curse. "Thorns and snares are in the way of the froward: he that doth keep his soul shall be far from them" (Proverbs 22:5).

We can spare ourselves the sorrows of the curse by not sowing among thorns. We are rewarded for that which we sow. "Be not deceived; God is not mocked: for whatsoever a man soweth, that shall he also reap" (Galatians 6:7). Thus, our reward is not only stored up in heavenly places, but we are reaping it even now. God has set the principles of life and death (blessings and curses) within the earth. He has given every one the free will to choose, but He entreats us to choose life and not death, blessings and not curses. We reward ourselves by reaping today what we sowed yesterday, whether good or bad. As we live for God and sow in the Spirit, we reap the fruit of our reward and will continue to reap through out eternity.

The wicked worketh a deceitful work: but to him that soweth righteousness shall be a sure reward.
—Proverbs 11:18

Prayer

Heavenly Father, thank You for Your great faithfulness—I know You work all things, even pain, brokenness, and suffering together for the good of those who love You. Reveal to me the unique and awesome purpose You have planned for my life and make me strong in my weaknesses through Your power and truth. Help me to choose life in every decision I make. In Jesus' name, Amen!

15

A Day in God's Courts:
Better than a Thousand Elsewhere

*For a day in thy courts is better than a thousand. I
had rather be a doorkeeper in the house of my God,
than to dwell in the tents of wickedness.*
—Psalm 84:10

Oftentimes we forget how presently rewarding
it is to live for God, until we recall how far
He has brought us from the sour grapes of sin. For
the inner peace and security, which we have in the
Lord, provides a choice plum, far beyond worldly
pleasures. Having the presence of God in our lives
is priceless, beyond anything we could ever deserve.
Better is one day in His courts than a thousand else-
where (Psalm 84:10). Nothing compares to walking

in the anointing—in the manifest presence of God. Disobeying God is a massive mistake because we rob Him of His glory, and we stifle our storehouse of blessing. God is our life-sustaining and saving power. People, at some point, say they would give anything to receive a miracle. Just give your life, your heart to Jesus Christ. He is the miracle worker in the earth and there is no greater miracle than salvation. Man can't do what God can do. He's always right there when we need Him. And in the midst of life trials and world crises such as illness, persecution, war and catastrophic events, it's great to know that the Lord is on your side (Psalm 118:6). The children of Israel realized it when they were abiding safe in Goshen, while plagues and destruction visited the Egyptians (Exodus 8:22). Likewise, the Ark of God brought blessings upon Obed-Edom's house (2 Samuel 6:11), but upon the Philistines, it broke idols, destroyed the people, and smote many with hemorrhoids (1 Samuel 5:4-7). Israel knew that having the Ark of the Covenant with them in battle was the key to their victory.

Furthermore, the glorious temple in the center of Jerusalem represented their prosperity and safety. Without it, protection, joy, and unity diminished. Likewise, our lives depend upon having God in the center. We have the opportunity to invest time, instead of wasting it, by relishing in God's presence and making Him the center of our lives. Nothing is of greater benefit to us than seeking God's face. God offers us protection from evil. In Psalm 27, David's life example reveals what happens when you seek

God first. In times of trouble, the Lord will hide you in His shelter and set you high upon a rock of safety above your enemies. He'll give you confidence and you will see His goodness. This revelation is due to David's obedience and pursuit of intimacy with God and is relevant for those confiding in God today. There's no substitute for making God priority. Overcoming the pain of persecution and other heartaches takes a commitment from us to seek God's face, and a deep, yearning thirst after Him the way the parched deer pants for the water brooks. Divine deliverance is yours when you're walking with God's power; trusting in His salvation. David said that he would have fainted unless he had believed to see the goodness of the Lord in the land of the living (Psalm 27:13). As we spend time in God's presence, He imparts divine hope so that we don't lose heart and doubt His purposes for our lives. His presence yields peaceable fruits of righteousness, and results in great dividends of joy and contentment. He is worth living for and He is our greatest reward.

Brethren, we desire something better than this world. Do you not? Has the world ever satisfied you? Perhaps it did when you were dead in sin. A dead world may satisfy a dead heart, but ever since you have known something of better things, have you ever been contented with this world?
—Charles Haddon Spurgeon

Prayer

Father, I want more of You in my life. I long for Your presence and Your power to fill me and envelop me. You satisfy my every thirst and every need. You are my portion O' Lord. Without You, I can do nothing (John 15:5).

Part 5
A Victim or Victor?
Live as an Overcomer

16

The Lame will Leap like a Hart

And he said unto me, My grace is sufficient for thee:
for my strength is made perfect in weakness. Most
gladly therefore will I rather glory in my infirmities,
that the power of Christ may rest upon me.
—2 Corinthians 12:9

While "lame" can mean *having a disabled limb*;
it can also simply mean *weak*. Lameness can
cause people to be despondent, preventing them from
fulfilling dreams and hopes for their lives. However,
in every weakness there is great spiritual potential!
There is potential that far exceeds our own human
capabilities. The potential is found in our weakness,
because it is there, through Christ, that we are made
strong. Christians should not focus on disadvantages,
but rather take advantage of opportunities to wax

strong through God's strength. Amazingly, weaknesses we tend to think will disqualify us can be the very things that miraculously qualify us to fulfill our purpose and destiny. In the book of Acts, we read of a lame man who was healed when Peter said, "In the name of Jesus Christ of Nazareth rise up and walk" (Acts 3:6b). Scripture tells us that the fellow did more than walk. For as his feet and ankle bones received strength, he went leaping and walking, praising God! Likewise, as we allow God's presence to manifest in our weakness, we will receive strength that will catapult us to new spiritual levels of progress. God's Spirit can enable us to leap over the barricading walls of our own insecurities and doubts, "by my God have I leaped over a wall" (2 Samuel 22:30b).

Through God's power, we can accomplish great exploits, far surpassing our own limited capabilities. The book of Isaiah prophesies that the lame will leap like a deer (35:6 NIV). Regardless of whether it's a physical or emotional weakness, this is an opportunity to leap into higher realms and levels of God, "He maketh my feet like hinds' feet: and setteth me upon my high places" (2 Samuel 22:34). We can be empowered spiritually to leap from glory to glory, strength to strength, and faith to faith. Even when we are suffering from persecution, Jesus instructed us to leap for joy, because our reward is great in heaven (Luke 6:23). Regardless of the cause, our affliction is working on our behalf.

For all things are for your sakes, that the abundant grace might through the thanksgiving of many redound to the glory of God. For which cause we faint not; but though our outward man perish, yet the inward man is renewed day by day. For our light affliction, which is but for a moment, worketh for us a far more exceeding and eternal weight of glory;—2 Corinthians 4:15–17

It is vain for us to glory in our own limited human capabilities (1 Corinthians 1:29), but we can glory in our tribulations because they are not working against us, but for us!

And not only so, but we glory in tribulations also: knowing that tribulation worketh patience; And patience, experience; and experience, hope: And hope maketh not ashamed;
—Romans 5:3-5a

Yes, we can leap for joy, knowing that weaknesses, afflictions, and tribulations are all sources for God's abilities to be wrought in us. For Paul wrote:

Therefore I take pleasure in infirmities, in reproaches, in necessities, in persecutions, in distresses for Christ's sake: for when I am weak, then am I strong.

—2 Corinthians 12:10

As we acknowledge our infirmities, we also acknowledge our need to rely upon God. Before Jacob could become a prince who prevails with God (Israel), the hollow of his thigh had to be put out of joint. Thus, he worshipped God, leaning upon his staff. Because Israel "halted upon his thigh" (Genesis 32:31), he shall leap for joy in these last days. God has ordained Israel, the seed of Abraham and the Bride of Christ, even the one that halteth to become a remnant and a spiritually strong nation (Micah 4:7).

Usually, it's only when we lose our own stability that we learn to lean upon God's strength. Blind Samson had to lean against pillars, but as he leaned, he prayed for the Lord to strengthen him. He then received his greatest strength, which enabled him to avenge his enemies. In the Song of Solomon there is one described as coming up from the wilderness leaning on her beloved (8:5a). She prophetically represents the Bride of Christ who relies and leans upon Jesus. The disciple who Scripture calls the one "whom Jesus loved" knew how to lean upon Jesus' bosom. For there truly is none other to lean upon but He who upholds all things by the word of His power (Hebrews 1:3). And as we lean upon Him we can be "strengthened with all might, according to his glorious power, unto all patience and longsuffering with joyfulness" (Colossians 1:11).

So rejoice as you rely upon Jesus for strength because God's strength becomes yours when you grab hold of the horns of the altar. If you are relying upon your own strength to carry you through life, you are destined to fall. Those who structure their lives according to the fallacious wisdom of this world are bound for disappointment. The Bible says that the wisdom of this world is foolishness with God, and it shall be brought to naught: "Let no man deceive himself. If any man among you seemeth to be wise in this world, let him become a fool, that he may be wise" (1 Corinthians 3:18). If you are foolish in the sight of the world, then perhaps, you are a prime candidate to receive God's strength. Only when we acknowledge our foolishness and weakness will we seek and rely on the wisdom that comes from above. The work of God that is wrought in our lives is greater than works of the flesh. God is glorified because our flesh has nothing to boast of itself. Rather, we know that our strength comes from God, and therefore He receives all the glory.

For ye see your calling, brethren, how that not many wise men after the flesh, not many mighty, not many noble, are called: But God hath chosen the foolish things of the world to confound the wise; and God hath chosen the weak things of the world to confound the things which are mighty; And base things of the world, and things which are despised, hath God chosen, yea, and things which are not, to bring to nought things that are: That no flesh should glory in his presence. But of him are ye in Christ Jesus, who of God is made unto us wisdom, and righteousness, and sanctification, and redemption: That, according as it is written, He that glorieth, let him glory in the Lord. — 1 Corinthians 1:26–31

God uses men and women who are weak, feeble,
and humble enough to lean on Him.
—Unknown

Prayer

Lord, You are my strength when I am weak and You are the treasure that I seek. You sent Your Son so that I can have life and life more abundantly (John 10:10). Father, the reason I live is to glorify You.

17

Divine Landings

Wherein ye greatly rejoice, though now for a season, if need be, ye are in heaviness through manifold temptations:
—1 Peter 1:6

Have you been thrown into a dark situation? If so, don't be too disheartened; you may find yourself in a divine landing. Satan enjoys casting God's children into dire predicaments and perilous situations. Joseph was thrown into the pit (Genesis 37:24). Daniel was thrown into the lions' den (Daniel 6:16). Shadrach, Meshach, and Abednego were thrown into the fiery furnace (Daniel 3:20). Paul and Silas were thrown into prison (Acts 16:24). Early century Christians were even thrown into bull pits. The list could go on, but Scripture reveals that the ultimate landings of their falls were in the hands of God.

Satan may throw Christians, but God uses that same throw, to throw worldly debris out of our lives. When the righteous are thrown, unrighteousness is often thrown off. Sometimes it takes us being thrown by the enemy before we will get serious enough with God to throw down idolatrous altars, unhealthy relationships, pride, prejudices and other obstacles that hinder our intimacy with God. Sometimes it takes a fire to burn away the ropes that bind us up.

You might be bound when you're thrown into the fire, but when you're in it, you can be loosed, just like Shadrach, Meshach and Abednego, because that's where you will get desperate and passionate enough to meet Jesus (Daniel 3:25). Joseph was thrown not only into the pit, but into prison as well. In both, he was proven as a faithful servant of the Lord, and he soon found himself landing at the throne of Pharaoh. One day of favor with the Lord is greater than a thousand days of labor. We need to keep in mind that God gives the increase and promotion comes from Him (Psalm 75:6,7).

Our faith in Christ should compel us to cling to the promises of God, rather than clinging to the problem. Anyone can succumb to discouragement by simply focusing on the trial, rather than the Word of God. We need to look to the spiritual realm and stand upon the promises of Almighty God. If we will turn our eyes to Jesus when thrown into dire predicaments, the Lord will take us from crisis to celebration as we land where He has destined.

A crisis, a trial—what a season to get into the Word of God like never before; to cry out to God, and praise Him with all of your heart, thanking Him for the victory that He won on your behalf and for manifesting His victory in your circumstance and situation.

Paul could rejoice through his major trials because He walked in the Spirit and the Word encouraged his heart. How else could he survive that dark dungeon of a prison (Acts 16:25)? He and Silas rejoiced and sang early in the morning, and they worshipped God right through discouragement.

We can also find encouragement in the Word of God, even in the hard times; especially since it reveals that God casts down the enemy. It tells us that God threw the Egyptians into the Red Sea (Exodus 14:27), and Jezebel to the street to be eaten by dogs (1 Kings 21:23). The book of Revelation reveals how judgment will cause Babylon to be thrown down (Revelation 18:21). And, yes, "the dragon, that old serpent, which is the Devil, and Satan" shall be thrown into the bottomless pit (Revelation 20:2, 3). God will have the last throw! It's better to be thrown into a crisis that results with a divine landing than to be thrown away from God's throne and His presence forevermore.

*When the devil and the world combine to persecute
a Christly soul, they put him on the throne of power.*
— G. Campbell Morgan

Prayer

Father, I praise You and know that all things work together for the good of those who love You, who are called according to Your purpose (Romans 8:28). I declare, "The right hand of the LORD is exalted: the right hand of the LORD doeth valiantly" (Psalm 118:16). I pray that I will fulfill the calling and purpose that You have for my life. I want to abide with You forever. In Jesus' name. Amen.

18

Lifted from the Ash Heap

O thou afflicted, tossed with tempest, and not comforted, behold, I will lay thy stones with fair colours, and lay thy foundations with sapphires.
—Isaiah 54:11

Throughout Scripture, we see many who were called of God and, as a result, they were afflicted, hated, despised. The Lord pities such people. But Scripture also reveals that God blesses and calls those who are already afflicted, hated and despised. He opened Leah's womb because He saw that she was hated (Genesis 29:31). God made Leah very fruitful. She named her first son Reuben, saying, "'Surely the LORD hath looked upon my affliction; now therefore my husband will love me'" (Genesis 29:32b). The second child she named Simeon, saying, "'Because the LORD hath heard that I was hated, he hath therefore given me this son also'" (Genesis 29:33b).

In First Corinthians it is written, "And base things of the world, and things which are despised, hath God chosen, yea, and things which are not, to bring to nought things that are" (1:28).

If you've been despised, rejected, or abused, don't pity yourself. Rather, you can let God pity you and favor you, and expect to receive God's strength and blessing. Even as God blessed Leah with the fruit of the womb, so you can be strengthened by God to bear the fruit of the Spirit.

But the fruit of the Spirit is love, joy, peace, longsuffering, gentleness, goodness, faith, —Galatians 5:22

What the enemy intends for evil, God turns for good in the lives of His people. "Behold, I have refined thee, but not with silver; I have chosen thee in the furnace of affliction" (Isaiah 48:10). Though certain people may have caused you much pain, a greater love can be rooted in your heart. As we give our lives to God and forgive the ones who severely hurt us, an unconditional love is wrought in our hearts. Otherwise we wouldn't be able to forgive those who have hurt us so badly. But because God commands us to forgive others, even as He forgives us, we have to allow the unconditional love of God to fill our wounds. After forgiving those who have intensely hurt us, we can truly say we know what it means to forgive others. And if we know forgiveness, we know love; even the love of God. Do you see how God uses the things and people that weakened you to ultimately strengthen you? The Bible says, "let the weak say, I am strong" (Joel 3:10b). There is no greater strength than the strength of God's love. Through God's love, fear becomes faith, intemperance becomes temperance, perversion becomes purity, and pride becomes humility.

Never wallow in self-pity, regardless of the hardship you may face. No matter how weak you are, rest assured that you have at least enough reserve to lean on Him. Allow God to do the pitying, and expect His favor and blessings. He will turn your poor mentality into a mindset of possession.

He raises the poor from the dust and lifts the needy from the ash heap; he seats them with princes and has them inherit a throne of honor.—1 Samuel 2:8 NIV

Don't let rejection or loneliness overtake you, but rather trust in God's Word that says, "God setteth the solitary in families: he bringeth out those which are bound with chains" (Psalm 68:6a). It also tell us that He hears the groans of the prisoners, and releases those who are condemned to death (Psalm 102:20 NIV).

The areas of your life where you have been victimized are the very areas in which you can be an incredible victor through Christ. Even the attacks of Satan that tear you down work out for God's glory, because those who are forgiven much will love much. God takes that which Satan has meant for evil and turns it for good. "But where sin abounded, grace did much more abound" (Romans 5:20b). There is weeping for a night in our dark sin, but there is joy in the morning as we see the light of God's forgiveness. David wept over his sin that resulted in the death of his son, but in the morning forgiveness shone in the birth of Solomon.

God truly wants His people to be comforted. The Holy Spirit is our Comforter in the world of tribulation. From persecutions to judgments, Jerusalem has experienced tremendous upheaval, turmoil and ruination. Likewise, the Body of Christ has shed much blood, sweat, and tears. Nevertheless, God is merciful and He is a restorer of the breach and a repairer of the broken. God will lay Jerusalem's stones with fair colors and her foundations with sapphires. Just as God will deck Jerusalem, so will He beautify His covenant people who have been afflicted, tossed with tempest and not comforted (Isaiah 54:11-13). Though Jesus warned of the tribulation we will have in the world, He called us to be of good cheer because He has overcome the world (John 16:33).

Thou hast caused men to ride over our heads;
we went through fire and through water: but thou
broughtest us out into a wealthy place.
—Psalm 66:12

Prayer
(Psalm 4)

Hear me when I call, O God of my righteousness: thou hast enlarged me when I was in distress; have mercy upon me, and hear my prayer. O ye sons of men, how long will ye turn my glory into shame? how long will ye love vanity, and seek after leasing? Selah. But know that the LORD hath set apart him that is godly for himself: the LORD will hear when I call unto him. Stand in awe, and sin not: commune with your own heart upon your bed, and be still. Selah. Offer the sacrifices of righteousness, and put your trust in the LORD. There be many that say, Who will shew us any good? LORD, lift thou up the light of thy countenance upon us. Thou hast put gladness in my heart, more than in the time that their corn and their wine increased. I will both lay me down in peace, and sleep: for thou, LORD, only makest me dwell in safety.

19

Crushed in Spirit

The LORD is nigh unto them that are of a broken heart; and saveth such as be of a contrite spirit.
— Psalm 34:18

Even as God has numbered the hairs on your head and not one shall fall to the ground without His acknowledgment, so it is with your tears.

God is near to those who are contrite. Contrition is an act of grieving. The Hebrew word for contrition is *dakka,* and it means crushed, bruised, and contrite. The Spirit of the Lord is attracted to those who are contrite. When we are exceedingly sorrowful, God often sends an angel to comfort us, just as He did for Jesus in the Garden of Gethsemane (Luke 22:43).

Perhaps, God does store up our tears before He pours out the answer to our cries (Psalm 56:8).

However, when He does pour it out, a flood of redemption accompanies the outpouring. For centuries, the children of Israel cried out for deliverance from their Egyptian oppressors, and finally the cup of their sufferings filled to the brim. The pain of their groans was seen and heard by YHWH the God of Abraham, the God of Isaac, and the God of Jacob and He came down to deliver His people. "I have seen, I have seen the affliction of my people which is in Egypt, and I have heard their groaning, and am come down to deliver them. And now come, I will send thee into Egypt" (Acts 7:34). At that point, God was ready to deliver the Hebrews, and from out of the burning bush, He called Moses. Nevertheless, the battle between Pharaoh and Moses grew increasingly intense, as did the sufferings of the Israelites who were beaten for their incomplete work. The more the cup of their cries overflowed, the more God intervened to bring judgment on Egypt, for their cries moved God to act. Likewise, He moves with the groaning of all His covenant children.

For thus saith the high and lofty One that inhabiteth eternity, whose name is Holy; I dwell in the high and holy place, with him also that is of a contrite and humble spirit, to revive the spirit of the humble, and to revive the heart of the contrite ones. — Isaiah 57:15

The prayers of the righteous are not in vain. God has always heard the cries of His people. He heard the cry of Jonah from the belly of the great fish and commanded the fish to vomit him out on to dry land (Jonah 2:2,10). He heard the cry of David and spared him from the sword of Saul (Psalm 18:6). He heard the cry of Hezekiah and healed him, adding fifteen more years to his life (2 Kings 20:5,6). "The righteous cry, and the LORD heareth, and delivereth them out of all their troubles" (Psalm 34:17).

There are more tears shed over answered prayers than over unanswered ones.
—Teresa of Avila

Prayer
(Psalm 56)

Be merciful unto me, O God: for man would swallow me up; he fighting daily oppresseth me. Mine enemies would daily swallow me up: for they be many that fight against me, O thou most High. What time I am afraid, I will trust in thee. In God I will praise his word, in God I have put my trust; I will not fear what flesh can do unto me. Every day they wrest my words: all their thoughts are against me for evil. They gather themselves together, they hide themselves, they mark my steps, when they wait for my soul. Shall they escape by iniquity? in thine anger cast down the people, O God. Thou tellest my wanderings: put thou my tears into thy bottle: are they not in thy book? When I cry unto thee, then shall mine enemies turn back: this I know; for God is for me. In God will I praise his word: in the LORD will I praise his word. In God have I put my trust: I will not be afraid what man can do unto me. Thy vows are upon me, O God: I will render praises unto thee. For thou hast delivered my soul from death: wilt not thou deliver my feet from falling, that I may walk before God in the light of the living?

20

Touched with Feelings that Hurt

For we have not an high priest which cannot be touched with the feeling of our infirmities; but was in all points tempted like as we are, yet without sin.
—Hebrews 4:15

Though God can relate to us through His omniscient discernment of our feelings and emotions, He still reached out to relate to us in our fleshly attire by sending His Son. "And the Word was made flesh, and dwelt among us" (John 1:14a). Jesus was touched with the same feelings that we experience. Of course, He is the reason why we as believers, experience many of the things we do.

Remember the word that I said unto you,
The servant is not greater than his lord. If they
have persecuted me, they will also persecute
you; if they have kept my saying, they will
keep yours also. But all these things will they
do unto you for my name's sake, because they
know not him that sent me. —John 15:20, 21

Jesus knows what it means to be despised and
rejected. He can empathize with your pain. Many
sufferings of people are not necessarily a direct
persecution, but a result of a demonic target against
the high calling of God. Often we demean the sufferings that Jesus endured, not knowing the extent of
His pain. But Scripture reveals that "his visage was
so marred more than any man, and his form more
than the sons of men" (Isaiah 52:14b). Of course
one of His greatest agonies was the grieving of His
heart as sinful men loved darkness rather than light.
He knows how it feels to be hated for no reason.
He knows how it feels to reach out with everything
within a heart's capacity for the goodwill and benefit
of others, only to be rejected, despised and abused.

In our times of misery, we are not alone, because
we have a great High Priest who can sympathize with
us in our pain; regardless if our pain is for the sake
of God or due to other evil tidings. Jesus has been
touched with the feelings of our infirmities (Hebrews
4:15). We are not to deny negative emotions caused
by hurt or sorrow; however, we must turn to God

and release them to the Lord and allow His love to embrace us. Jesus felt our pain, so that we might be able to feel others and through His Spirit, intercede for them.

I would rather feel compassion than know the meaning of it.
—Thomas Aquinas

Prayer
St. Francis of Assissi (1182-1226)

"LORD, make me an instrument of your peace. Where there is hatred, let me sow love; where there is injury, pardon; where there is doubt, faith; where there is despair, hope; where there is darkness, light; where there is sadness, joy. O Divine Master, grant that I may not so much seek to be consoled as to console; to be understood as to understand; to be loved as to love. For it is in giving that we receive; it is in pardoning that we are pardoned; and it is in dying that we are born to eternal life."

Part 6
Intercessory Sufferings

21

Godly Sorrow:
Seeing our Sin in the Light of
His Love

For godly sorrow worketh repentance to salvation
not to be repented of: but the sorrow of the world
worketh death.
—2 Corinthians 7:10

Do you ever feel sorry about the great price that Jesus had to pay for your sins to be forgiven? As your eyes are open to the intense, brutal sufferings that Jesus experienced as your sins nailed Him to the cross, is there a sorrow that fills your heart? His suffering for us was so intense that "his appearance was so disfigured beyond that of any man and his form marred beyond human likeness" (Isaiah 52:14b NIV).

As we acknowledge Jesus' innocence and gain the revelation of His unconditional, sacrificial love, we see the stark reality of our sinful rebellion epitomized in our rejection of Him. Scripture reveals how Jesus was despised and rejected of men, a man of sorrows, and acquainted with grief (Isaiah 53:3). Realizing that God's own Son experienced sorrow for our sakes makes us sorrowful for our calloused hearts, which despised Him. Through revelation, we see that it was us—we who hid our faces from Him, and we no longer blame His death on the Roman soldiers or the religious Jews. While there is a bitter agony that fills our souls with sorrow, nevertheless we are eternally grateful for the price that He paid for our sins.

> and they shall look upon me whom they
> have pierced, and they shall mourn for him,
> as one mourneth for his only son, and shall be
> in bitterness for him, as one that is in bitter-
> ness for his firstborn.—Zechariah 12:10b

This is a good sorrow, different from the sorrow of the world. "For godly sorrow worketh repentance to salvation not to be repented of: but the sorrow of the world worketh death" (2 Corinthians 7:10). Only when we are truly sorry for our sins will we repent of them. Incorrigible hearts don't have sorrow over sin, only pliable hearts can beat with God's love.

As Jesus bore the cross on His way to Calvary, a great company of people followed, wailing and lamenting Him. "But Jesus turning unto them said, Daughters of Jerusalem, weep not for me, but weep for yourselves, and for your children" (Luke 23:28). Jesus did not imply that we shouldn't have remorse over our sins, and regret the pain and suffering that He had to endure for us; as our sins nailed Him to the cross. Instead, He was saying to weep because of the judgment that is coming in these last days. As we weep and cry out to God in repentance, our reward will come in deliverance from wrath and destruction. God spared Nineveh from His fierce wrath because the people cried out in repentance (Jonah 3:8–10). The Jews were able to protect themselves from their enemies through Esther's petition of the king after they greatly mourned, wept, and wailed unto the Lord (Esther 4:3). As we return unto the Lord and cry out in repentance, our reward will be a blessing instead of a curse.

Let the priests, the ministers of the LORD, weep between the porch and the altar, and let them say, Spare thy people, O LORD, and give not thine heritage to reproach, that the heathen should rule over them:… Yea, the LORD will answer and say unto his people,

Behold, I will send you corn, and wine, and oil, and ye shall be satisfied therewith: and I will no more make you a reproach among the heathen: —Joel 2:17a-19

Do you have godly sorrow because God's Word is not obeyed and His presence loved and adored? The Psalmist who loved the Lord did: "Rivers of waters run down mine eyes, because they keep not thy law" (Psalm 119:136). Many of the prophets did, including Samuel, who cried all night unto the Lord when he was grieved by Saul's disobedience (1 Samuel 15:11). Jeremiah said his heart was broken within him because of the prophets who were disobedient to God (23:9).

Do you have godly sorrow for those who are living in sin and will face severe judgments, unless they repent? The Apostle Paul spoke of bewailing those who sinned and did not repent of their fornication and lasciviousness (2 Corinthians 12:21).

Do you have the heartbeat of God to cry out for others? As you intercede and cry out for the lost, you are saving others with fear, pulling them out of the fire (Jude 23). They might not be saved yet, but don't grow weary. You can count on divine assurance that your tears are not in vain! Your reward will be the joy of the harvest, as you usher the lost into the presence of the Lord. "He that goeth forth and weepeth, bearing precious seed, shall doubtless come again with rejoicing, bringing his sheaves with him" (Psalm 126:6).

From Scripture we can know that having godly sorrow is a reward in itself. This is because it manifests such great things in us. It clears us, through repentance, from our guilt and carnal ways. Godly sorrow puts the indignation of the Lord in us by awakening us to the reality that God detests sin. Righteous indignation is aroused against Satan and his cohorts. This awakens us to the fact that the devil is real, not just a mere cartoon character, but a diabolical spirit that can be addressed in the spirit realm with the authority of Christ. We realize the intensity of the spiritual battle for the souls of mankind and therefore, we become valiant in fight, relying on spiritual weapons of faith and the Word of God to overcome. Godly sorrow causes us to begin with wisdom in the reverential fear of the Lord. It stirs us up in a vehement desire for holiness and purity wherein we refuse to keep repeating the same sins, like a dog returning to its own vomit. Godly sorrow manifests a zeal and boldness to proclaim the Gospel to others. It births in us the desire to please God, rather than conform to society. It breathes a desire for revenge against all ungodliness and unrighteousness. The true essence of our hatefulness toward sin is proved by the intensity of our desire for deliverance, whether for our selves or others. This desire fosters a holy jealousy, which is expressed in desperate acts of intercession: "And having in a readiness to revenge all disobedience, when your obedience is fulfilled" (2 Corinthians 10:6). This passion stirs our hearts to cry out for ourselves and to intercede for others, that we may snatch them from the fire and save them (Jude 23).

Do you think we could sit still, or grow worldly, or spend all our energies upon ourselves, if we could see the Crucified One? Faith, when it stands at the foot of the cross, makes us hate sin and love the Savior just as much as though we had seen our sins placed to Christ's account, and had seen the nails driven through his hands and feet, and seen the bloody scourges as they made the sacred drops of blood to fall.
—Charles Haddon Spurgeon

Prayer

Father God, I want to put every sinful desire to death—I pray that You will birth in me a hatred for sin and ungodliness. Create in me a pure heart and renew a steadfast spirit within me. Unite my heart to fear You and follow You. Help me to see sin as You see it, and to hate it as You hate it. I pray that You will give me Your heart for those who are lost, that I might cry out for them. Lord, birth in me a passion to intercede for those who do not know You. In Jesus' name. Amen

22

Preserving Life:
The Gain of our Pain through
Intercession

They that sow in tears shall reap in joy.
—Psalm 126:5

The biblical account of the life of Joseph illustrates the life of the Messiah. Joseph endured many intercessory sufferings. His brothers were jealous of their father's great love for him. Thus, they cast him into a pit and sold him to Midianite merchants who carried him away to Egypt. Years later, Joseph was able to see his brethren again, and at that time, God fulfilled Joseph's childhood dreams. Nevertheless, when Joseph revealed himself to his brethren, they were troubled at his presence.

However, Joseph comforted them and said that God sent him to Egypt to preserve life: "Now therefore be not grieved, nor angry with yourselves, that ye sold me hither: for God did send me before you to preserve life" (Genesis 45:5). God used Joseph to prepare Egypt for a seven-year period of famine. Because the famine was also in the land of Canaan, Joseph's brethren came to Egypt seeking provision. Joseph, who was exalted as ruler throughout Egypt, saved his family's lives by a great deliverance. He explained, "And God sent me before you to preserve you a posterity in the earth, and to save your lives by a great deliverance" (Genesis 45:7).

Joseph was not bitter about all the sufferings he had to endure, because he knew that God had a plan for his life and a reason for him being in Egypt. He knew that they were intercessory sufferings. He knew that he suffered for the sake of the salvation of others, including the very ones who afflicted him, but not only for them, but for the sake of many to come (future generations). Because Joseph's life was a prophetic type of Christ's, it also serves as a prophetic type of the lives of Christ's followers. Just as Jesus was crucified for the salvation and preservation of others, so we are appointed to intercessory sufferings. "And they that are Christ's have crucified the flesh with the affections and lusts" (Galatians 5:24).

Like Joseph, you may be rejected, despised, falsely accused, abandoned, or confined. However, just as Joseph's sufferings were not in vain, neither are yours, in as much as they are for the Lord. There's a plan of God in motion, as you suffer for Christ's sake. The pain that you endure for the sake of Christ, is reaching heaven through cries that are preserving life for others. The prayers of the saints are offered, with incense, upon the golden altar before the throne of God (Revelation 8:3). When you truly see the gain of your pain, you won't ever regret any loss.

The passion that the Lord births in our hearts for the salvation of others will result in rewards that far outweigh our afflictions. Our suffering lasts only for this life, but is preserving and saving lives for eternity: "And he that reapeth receiveth wages, and gathereth fruit unto life eternal: that both he that soweth and he that reapeth may rejoice together" (John 4:36).

Only God knows the multitudes that your life impacts as you worship, witness, give, and pray. Yes, these all entail self denial and intercessory sufferings, but reap great rewards.

At the cross, the disciples did not know the salvation that was being ushered into the world. Likewise, we often don't know the extent of the salvation that is being orchestrated in the spirit realm as we endure pain in Christ's name. But as God was faithful to Joseph, so will He fulfill His plan for your life as you trust and surrender to Him. Then you will see that God has sent you to preserve life and to save many through a great deliverance. Surely, your God-inspired dreams will be fulfilled as you carry in the sheaves (the harvest of your prayers).

The ultimate intercessory sufferings were, of course, experienced by Jesus who died for the sins of the world.

But he was wounded for our transgressions, he was bruised for our iniquities: the chastisement of our peace was upon him; and with his stripes we are healed. All we like sheep have gone astray; we have turned every one to his own way; and the LORD hath laid on him the iniquity of us all. He was oppressed, and he was afflicted, yet he opened not his mouth: he is brought as a lamb to the slaughter, and as a sheep before her shearers is dumb, so he openeth not his mouth. He was taken from prison and from judgment: and who shall declare his generation? for he was cut off out of the land of the living: for the transgression of my people was he stricken. And he made his grave with the wicked, and with the rich in his death; because he had done no violence, neither was any deceit in his mouth. Yet it pleased the LORD to bruise him; he hath put him to grief: when thou shalt make his soul an offering for sin, he shall see his seed, he shall prolong his days, and the pleasure of the LORD shall prosper in his hand.—Isaiah 53:5-10

When Jesus sees the travail of His soul, He is satisfied. He doesn't regret the pain He endured, because He was sent to preserve life and save many through a great deliverance. Through His pain, He has justified many.

Before His death, Jesus confessed His sacrifice for others in prayer: "And for their sakes I sanctify myself, that they also might be sanctified through the truth" (John 17:19). Jesus set Himself apart and abstained from carnality for our sakes. Sanctification requires self denial. Because of Jesus' intercessory sufferings, we are born again. And we, who are born again, are also called to stand in the gap for others through heart-felt intercession. We are called to painful intercessory sufferings in order for others to be born again. This requires sacrificing our own will to meet the needs of others. Jesus demonstrated this type of sacrifice in both His living and in His dying. God is asking us to let Him do it again through us today. Will you answer the call?

Some missionaries bound for Africa were laughed at by the boat captain. "You'll only die over there," he said. But a missionary replied, "Captain, we died before we started."
—Vance Havner

Prayer

Lord, like a rose trampled on the ground You took the pain for my sake. Lord, give me Your heart to cry out for others so that they will see the light of Your truth and Your saving power. We need You, Lord, more than anything else this world could ever offer.

23

Sacrificial Passion

For I could wish that myself were accursed from
Christ for my brethren, my kinsmen according
to the flesh:
—Romans 9:3

Moses had a sacrificial passion for Israel to be saved from God's wrath. He pleaded with God to forgive the people's sins and said, "Yet now, if thou wilt forgive their sin—; and if not, blot me, I pray thee, out of thy book which thou hast written" (Exodus 32:32). Paul had this same passion for Israel. He was exceedingly sorrowful, even unto death. He wished his life could be substituted for his brethren's knowledge of Christ. Paul wasn't accursed as he so asked, but his sacrificial life surely resulted and is resulting in the salvation of his brethren.

"Intercession" really means to stand between, and intercessory prayer is more than just a recital of names. When we pray for others, we enter into the whole sphere of suffering and pain by bringing before God the deepest needs of the suffering person. We carry these needs into the sphere of the healing work of Christ. What we seek to do in intercession is to confront the destructive forces of evil with the redemptive power that flowed from the suffering of Jesus upon the cross: "and with his stripes we are healed" (Isaiah 53:5b). Intercession is therefore a ministry of great importance, which works at a deep level of reality and confronts the pain and anguish of others with the victorious love of Jesus Christ.

Paul is a prime example of an intercessory sufferer. He agonized in birth for many. He referred to himself as a "father" in his letter to the Christians in Corinth. "My little children, of whom I travail in birth again until Christ be formed in you" (Galatians 4:19). In order to birth them into the kingdom, Paul and other apostles had to endure much suffering on their behalf. They were fools for Christ's sake, so that their brethren could be wise in Christ. They were weak, so that fellow Christians could be strong. They were despised, so that others could be honorable. The intercessory sufferings of Paul and other apostles included going hungry, thirsty, naked, and homeless. They were buffeted, reviled, persecuted and defamed. Furthermore, they became the filth of the world and the offscourging of all things (1 Corinthians 4:10-13). Paul considered these intercessory sufferings to be a privilege because he knew his spiritual children were his crown, joy, and fruit to his heavenly account. "For though ye have ten thousand instructors in Christ, yet have ye not many fathers: for in Christ Jesus I have begotten you through the gospel" (1 Corinthians 4:15). Likewise, our intercessory sufferings are not in vain, because they are working life in others. As you sanctify yourself by abstaining from fleshly lusts, others are being sanctified through your prayers and witness.

Wherefore Jesus also, that he might sanctify the people with his own blood, suffered without the gate. Let us go forth therefore unto him without the camp, bearing his reproach.—Hebrews 13:12, 13

Jesus identified with our finitude and pain. At the center of all prayer is Jesus, and especially of intercessory prayer. Jesus waits for us, calling us to follow Him, praying for the oppressed, just as He prayed for us. We may not know the exact needs, but as we approach God in faith, the Holy Spirit will guide us in intercession. Through the love of God, we can identify with the pain of others and intercede on their behalf.

There is a place where thou canst touch the eyes
Of blinded men to instant, perfect sight;
There is a place where thou canst say, "Arise"
To dying captives, bound in chains of night;
There is a place where thou canst reach the store
Of hoarded gold and free it for the Lord;
There is a place—upon some distant shore—
Where thou canst send the worker and the Word.
Where is that secret place—dost thou ask,
"Where?"
O soul, it is the secret place of prayer!
—Alfred, Lord Tennyson

As you endure afflictions for Christ's sake, His kingdom is advancing in the earth and many are coming to salvation. In the book of Philippians, Paul spoke of his chains abounding to the spreading of the Gospel (1:12). Like Paul's, our sufferings for the Lord are abounding to our spiritual account. As we continue to intercede and cry out for the restoration of God's kingdom, we are bound to see the fullness of our callings unfold and more souls ushered into the saving power of God's presence—-all of which we will celebrate throughout eternity.

If sinners be damned, at least let them leap to Hell over our bodies. If they will perish, let them perish

with our arms about their knees. Let no one GO
there UNWARNED and UNPRAYED for.
—Charles Haddon Spurgeon

Prayer

Father, break me for the nations—let my life become Your light to all the world. I pray that You will send me to the lost, as an ambassador, to speak Your Holy Word. Lord, like bread that is broken, use my life and like wine that is poured forth, let me be a living sacrifice. Let my life count for all eternity. In Jesus' name, I pray. Amen.

24

Moved Enough to Weep

Remember them that are in bonds, as bound with them; and them which suffer adversity, as being yourselves also in the body.
—Hebrews 13:3

Intercessory sufferings are experienced in the spirit realm when we empathize with the pain of others and agonize in prayer for them. Just as our reproach fell upon Jesus, so we bear the burden of others through intense intercession. God wants us to engage in such deep and passionate intercession wherein our cries become so intense that we're grasping souls and claiming their salvation! As Jesus' soul was exceedingly sorrowful even unto death, so should ours be for others who are desperately in need of God's intervention. "Let us go forth therefore unto him without the camp, bearing his reproach" (Hebrews 13:13). Sometimes we don't immediately see the fruit of our labor, but its coming.

꧁꧂

> But whereunto shall I liken this genera-tion? It is like unto children sitting in the markets, and calling unto their fellows, And saying, We have piped unto you, and ye have not danced; we have mourned unto you, and ye have not lamented. —Matthew 11:16, 17

Christians are intercessory sufferers of one another. Intercession starts with the function of the Body of Christ, which means if one member hurts, the other members feel the pain. We suffer with each other and we suffer for one another. "And whether one member suffer, all the members suffer with it; or one member be honoured, all the members rejoice with it" (1 Corinthians 12:26). As a body, we suffer together. There is an endurance and comfort in knowing that you are not suffering alone, and a confidence to resist the enemy. "Whom resist sted-fast in the faith, knowing that the same afflictions are accomplished in your brethren that are in the world" (1 Peter 5:9). The apostle John called himself a companion in tribulation with other Christians (notice how he relates it to the Kingdom Principle):

꧁꧂

I John, who also am your brother, and companion in tribulation, and in the kingdom and patience of Jesus Christ, was in the isle that is called Patmos, for the word of God, and for the testimony of Jesus Christ.

—Revelation 1:9

Prayer sessions are not solely for self-edification. The Holy Spirit can prompt us to pray for our brothers and sisters in Christ who are in need, as well as for the lost. If God's love is at work in you, you will care about others, and your love for them will lead you to take it to the ultimate source of love.

We never really pray alone. When the true love inside of you for others moves you to ask God to act: to heal, strengthen, deliver, or transform another, the Holy Spirit is there praying through you. The Spirit leads you to pray and draws you into it.

We are to pray listening for the Spirit, because we don't always know what to pray. Someone may be hurting, hungry, or in danger. The Spirit will direct our prayer as we take heed to the promptings. When you intercede, you are allowing your passion and love for God to be used of Him; to operate and flow in the gifts of the Spirit, on behalf of others. If you find intercession hard, worship and meditate on Jesus and the Spirit will stir you with a desire to cry out for others.

The best prayers often have more groans than words.
—John Bunyan

Prayer

Father, give me a hatred for sin, but a love for the sinner and a heart for the hurting. Give me a desire to pray for those who are abused, sick, poor and others who need deliverance. Make me sensitive to Your Holy Spirit that I may be prompted to intercede and cry out as a companion in tribulation. Lord, instill in me Your love and compassion. Open the eyes of my heart's understanding and compel me to deep intercession for Body of Christ and the lost.

25

House of Mourning

Blessed are they that mourn:
for they shall be comforted.
—Matthew 5:4

Solomon, whom God gave exceeding wisdom, is generally credited to writing the book of Ecclesiastes which claims that it is better to go to a house of mourning than to a house of feasting (Ecclesiastes 7:2). It also reveals that the heart of the wise is in the house of mourning, but the heart of fools is in the house of mirth (Ecclesiastes 7:4).

The Holy Spirit is our Comforter (John 14:16), and He comforts those who mourn, especially those who mourn for righteousness' sake. It should not be a rare thing for Christians to mourn. It has always been appropriate for people to mourn over the dead. And

Christians know that the dead are not just those who have died physically, but those who are separated from God. Therefore, Christians are to mourn for the spiritually dead and for the sins that bring death whether they are our own, those of our peers or the sins of the nations. "For the wages of sin is death; but the gift of God is eternal life through Jesus Christ our Lord" (Romans 6:23).

By mourning and lamenting our sins and the sins of others, we are humbling ourselves in the sight of the Lord, and He shall lift us up (James 4:10). But those who refuse to humble their souls before God and relish in their own fancies will soon find themselves mourning in regret of their hedonism. "Woe unto you that laugh now! for ye shall mourn and weep" (Luke 6:25b). The Bible reveals that many who lived luxuriously with the spirit of the world (Babylon) shall wail and lament. "And the merchants of the earth shall weep and mourn over her" (Revelation 18:11a).

The righteous mourn not only the deaths of others, but also their own demise. It can be painful to suppress fleshly cravings, but those who are in Christ are called to mortify the deeds of the flesh (Colossians 3:5). Regardless of whether suffering is a consequence of righteousness or unrighteousness, it can still bring us to a greater surrender and self-denial if we will grasp the opportunity to turn toward God.

While Jesus was on the earth, the disciples of John the Baptist came to Him questioning why Jesus' disciples did not fast as they did. "And Jesus said unto them, Can the children of the bridechamber mourn, as long as the bridegroom is with them?" (Matthew 9:15a). However, before Jesus departed from the earth, He prepared His disciples by saying, "Verily, verily, I say unto you, That ye shall weep and lament, but the world shall rejoice" (John 16:20a). Now that Jesus has ascended to the right hand of the throne of the Father, we mourn. We weep and lament in a fallen world; mourning and longing for the fullness of our Bridegroom's redemption. The hardships, persecutions, and afflictions that we face, at times, can leave us writhing in agony—pain that is indescribable as it cuts to the core of our hearts. It's in these times that we can only endure as we rely upon God's Spirit and stand upon His promises, knowing that He was put to the ultimate test of pain and endured for the joy that was set before Him.

But at His appearing not only us, but all the nations of the earth shall mourn.

Behold, he cometh with clouds; and every eye shall see him, and they also which pierced him: and all kindreds of the earth shall wail because of him. Even so, Amen.
—Revelation 1:7

While our Bridegroom is away, we are not left without. We have the Holy Spirit which is our Comforter. And we receive manifold return on things we give up for Jesus' name's sake. As we give up our voluptuous ways and pick up our cross, we soon discover that the joy outweighs the burden. Jesus' yoke is easy and His burden is light (Matthew 11:30). As we seek Him and continue to trust in Him, we also find our mourning is turned into dancing. "Thou hast turned for me my mourning into dancing: thou hast put off my sackcloth, and girded me with gladness" (Psalm 30:11). The Word of God tells us that there is a time to mourn and a time to dance (Ecclesiastes 3:4). The more we have experienced the former, the greater anointing we will have to exchange the former for the latter and will be able to share this joy with others, "To appoint unto them that mourn in Zion, to give unto them beauty for ashes, the oil of joy for mourning, the garment of praise for the spirit of heaviness" (Isaiah 61:3a).

Where are the marks of the cross in your life? Are there any points of identification with your Lord? Alas, too many Christians wear medals but carry no scars.
— Vance Havner

Prayer
(Psalm 130)

Out of the depths have I cried unto thee, O LORD. Lord, hear my voice: let thine ears be attentive to the voice of my supplications. If thou, LORD, shouldest mark iniquities, O Lord, who shall stand? But there is forgiveness with thee, that thou mayest be feared. I wait for the LORD, my soul doth wait, and in his word do I hope. My soul waiteth for the Lord more than they that watch for the morning: I say, more than they that watch for the morning. Let Israel hope in the LORD: for with the LORD there is mercy, and with him is plenteous redemption. And he shall redeem Israel from all his iniquities.

Part 7
Ascend! Ascend!

26
Humility Exalts

*Humble yourselves therefore under the mighty hand
of God, that he may exalt you in due time:*
·—1 Peter 5:6

Amyriad of circumstances and situations can
humble us, but Scripture encourages us to
humble ourselves. Because humility relates to lowliness, people tend to associate it with deprivation.
However, rather than relating to loss, it applies more
to gain, increase and promotion in God's kingdom.
Pride, the opposite of humility, leads to destruction
and a haughty spirit can cause one to fall (Proverbs
16:18). The spirit of pride caused Lucifer to fall from
heaven and to turn from light to darkness (Isaiah
14:12-15). Pride causes one to fall harder and much
lower than what God desires us to experience through
humility. The truth is that we can spare ourselves

much suffering by humbling ourselves before the Lord. Not only can we spare ourselves afflictions, but also through our humility, we are setting ourselves up to be exalted.

For this is a Kingdom Principle: "Humble yourselves in the sight of the Lord, and he shall lift you up" (James 4:10). No matter how low you feel, you should not allow your status to be one of inferiority, but rather humility. The world encourages promotion of self through climbing the ladder of success. However, in God's kingdom the ladder of ascent is revealed to covenant children who are lowly or bowed down. Because Jesus descended to the depths of the earth, He also ascended higher than all the heavens (Ephesians 4:10). Because of Jesus' humility and obedience unto death, He now has been given a name above every name in heaven, on the earth and below the earth (Philippians 2:8-10). When the disciples asked Jesus who was the greatest in the kingdom of heaven, He answered by setting a little child in the midst of them. "And said, Verily I say unto you, Except ye be converted, and become as little children, ye shall not enter into the kingdom of heaven" (Matthew 18:3). Jesus taught this same principle to His disciples after the mother of Zebedee's children asked that her sons be allowed to sit on Jesus' right and left hand in His kingdom.

But Jesus called them unto him, and said, Ye know that the princes of the Gentiles exercise dominion over them, and they that are great exercise authority upon them. But it shall not be so among you: but whosoever will be great among you, let him be your minister; And whosoever will be chief among you, let him be your servant: — Matthew 20:25–27

Jesus expounded on this principle by differentiating the humble with the ways of the Pharisees who sought recognition and promotion by men. He said that the Pharisees loved the uppermost seats in the synagogues and to be called by man, "Master." Jesus accentuated that exaltation in the kingdom does not come through self promoting tactics but rather comes through humility.

But he that is greatest among you shall be your servant. And whosoever shall exalt himself shall be abased; and he that shall humble himself shall be exalted.
                                                    —Matthew 23:11,12

Our Lord also told a parable about how men choose out the chief rooms. Those who choose the chief rooms are likely to be asked to move to a lower state, but those who choose the lowest rooms are likely to be bidden to go up higher. Through this parable, He revealed that whosoever exalts himself will be abased, but he who humbles himself will be exalted. This is a consistent biblical principle (Luke 14:8-11). Your humility will propel your spiritual progress. For example, when a tower is built, the higher the tower, the further down has to be dug. Similarly, the farther one pulls back the string on a bow, the farther the arrow is going to propel forward. When you run into the circumstances of life that cause you go back or down, just know that this is your preparation to go ahead: "The LORD upholdeth all that fall, and raiseth up all those that be bowed down" (Psalm 145:14). The more you bow and surrender areas of your life, the higher you can ascend into your calling and destiny. Scripture encourages Christians not to grow weary in well-doing, because in due time you will reap if you do not faint (Galatians 6:9). Due time can represent the time of a baby's delivery and is symbolic of your calling and destiny. To explain, through humility, the spiritual stature of Christ is being formed in you and at the time of maturity, you will see the fullness of your calling come forth. You may already be reaping rewards through your humility and are yet to reap more as the world approaches the delivery of the kingdom of God. Ultimately, your humility will catapult you into exaltation as you are resurrected in immortality to reign with Christ.

Humility is essential for the believer who aims to walk worthy in the Lord. Without it, we cannot grow. Without humility, we can never be like Jesus, "Take my yoke upon you, and learn of me; for I am meek and lowly in heart" (Matthew 11:29a). The book of Proverbs teaches that before honor is humility (15:33).

Self-exaltation, pride, and arrogance are all contrary to God's Spirit. Proverbs 22:4 says, "By humility and the fear of the LORD are riches, and honour, and life." The book of James reveals "God resisteth the proud, but giveth grace unto the humble" (4:6b).

It's easy to become focused on position and status, hoping to receive proper recognition. But even if you feel like you are on a backburner; engulfed in obscurity and others are raised to recognition and success faster than you; keep in mind that God is ultimately in control:

For promotion cometh neither from the east, nor from the west, nor from the south. But God is the judge: he putteth down one, and setteth up another—Psalm 75:6, 7

Scripture tells us that God's recognition counts more than human praise. God is able and willing to bless us according to His own timing. Obey God regardless of your present circumstances. In His good time, in this life, or perhaps the next, He will lift you up, you can count on that.

A truly humble man is sensible of his natural distance from God; of his dependence on Him; of the insufficiency of his own power and wisdom; and that it is by God's power that he is upheld and provided for, and that he needs God's wisdom to lead and guide him, and His might to enable him to do what he ought to do for Him.
—Jonathan Edwards

Prayer

Father, I come before You humbly and submissively asking You to forgive me of pride. Instead of focusing on myself, help me to remember Your love, Your grace, and Your incredible mercy. Help me to always desire what pleases You, and what will glorify Your name. Lord, it's all about You—it's all about You, Lord. I know that my life is like a vapor, here for just a moment (James 4:14). I acknowledge Your sovereignty and ask You to reign in my life. In Jesus' name. Amen.

27

Patience:
An Avenue for God's Power

For ye have need of patience, that, after ye have done the will of God, ye might receive the promise.
—Hebrews 10:36

Patience is another word for longsuffering, and may be better described as love's longsuffering. Your longsuffering is what enables you to possess your soul. Your suffering is for your gain. The way you possess your soul is the same way to possess everything else God intends for you to possess. The way is through patience. "In your patience possess ye your souls" (Luke 21:19). That's how Abraham obtained God's promise of blessing and multiplication

(Hebrews 6:15). For it is through patience, mixed with faith, that saints inherit the promises of God.

God allowed Job to go through a time of affliction, but afterwards He prolifically blessed him. We also at times face hardships, but it's through suffering that our characters are molded, shaped, and proven. Paul knew this and that's why he gloried in tribulations.

> And not only so, but we glory in tribulations also: knowing that tribulation worketh patience; And patience, experience; and experience, hope: And hope maketh not ashamed; because the love of God is shed abroad in our hearts by the Holy Ghost which is given unto us. — Romans 5:3-5

Suffering refines our character: In the book of Ecclesiastes, we read, "Sorrow is better than laughter, because a sad face is good for the heart" (7:3). Isn't it in times of suffering that you evaluate your life and consider your ways? It was in times of suffering that David vowed to God what he would and wouldn't do. "I will go into thy house with burnt offerings: I will pay thee my vows, Which my lips have uttered, and my mouth hath spoken, when I was in trouble" (Psalm 66:13, 14). The Psalmist said, "Before I was afflicted I went astray: but now have I kept thy word" (Psalm 119:67). As fire refines silver and gold, so fiery trials and tribulations can refine our characters, purging out the impurities, and transforming us into the likeness of Christ's character.

We possess our souls unto life as we allow God's Spirit to reign in us and we bear forth the fruit of the Spirit. Longsuffering is a fruit of the Spirit and one that stimulates the growth of other fruits of the Spirit. The trying of our faith works patience within us, so that we may mature in the likeness of Christ.

Patience is an avenue for God's power (2 Corinthians 12:12). The book of Revelation reveals the longsuffering of the saints as obedience and faith in Jesus Christ (14:12). As our characters are transformed to be more like Jesus, we have hope for the future of our callings and destinies. The Bible says that if we see it, then it's not hope; but if we don't see it, then we have to wait with patience for what we hope (Romans 8:24, 25). Our wait is not in vain. Our patience is not in vain because we know that God has glorious things prepared for us. "For since the beginning of the world men have not heard, nor perceived by the ear, neither hath the eye seen, O God, beside thee, what he hath prepared for him that waiteth for him" (Isaiah 64:4).

Even when it seems to be a long stretch of time for certain promises of God to unfold, there is no use wallowing in self-pity or complaining and we certainly won't expedite our divine destinies by turning back, so rather, we are called to remain steadfast and press ahead.

Though we suffer long in Christ, we grow strong in faith. Ultimately, we are waiting for the redemption of our bodies. "For our light affliction, which is but for a moment, worketh for us a far more exceeding and eternal weight of glory" (2 Corinthians 4:17).

Scripture admonishes us to run with patience the race that is set before us (Hebrews 12:1). Running with patience seems awfully paradoxical, but actually refers to having endurance. Jesus told the parable of the sower who went out to sow his seed. Some fell by the wayside, some upon a rock, some among thorns, and the rest on good ground. Jesus explained to His disciples that the seed represents the Word of God. The places the seed fell represent those who hear the Word of God. Out of all the people who hear the Word of God, none endure except those who, in the parable, are planted in good ground. They endure because they keep the Word of God that they hear and bring forth fruit with patience (Luke 8:11-15).

It takes patience to endure the test of time: "But he that shall endure unto the end, the same shall be saved" (Matthew 24:13). If we lack attributes of the divine nature such as patience, then we have become nearsighted and cannot see afar off. Jesus was able to endure and despise the shame He faced because he looked ahead to the joy that was set before Him (Hebrews 12:1). Now He sits at the right hand of the throne of God, never to regret the suffering He endured, but rejoicing because of it. There is a great recompense of reward for those who endure! God promises that blessed is the believer who perseveres under trial and stands the test, because that person will receive the crown of life that God has promised to those who love Him (James 1:12).

We have need of patience with ourselves and with others; with those below and those above us, and with our own equals; with those who love us and those who love us not; for the greatest things and for the least; against sudden inroads of trouble, and under daily burdens; against disappointments as to the weather, or the breaking of the heart; in the weariness of the body, or the wearing of the soul; in our own failure of duty, or others' failure towards us; in every-day wants, or in the aching of sickness or the decay of old age; in disappointment, bereavement, losses, injuries, reproaches; in heaviness of the heart, or its sickness amid delayed hopes. In all these things, from childhood's little troubles to the martyr's sufferings, patience is the grace of God, whereby we endure evil for the love of God.
—Edward B. Pusey (1800-1882)

Prayer

Father, I will wait for You and Your purposes to unfold in my life. Deepen my trust in You, Lord, to endure while I wait, to press in and press on in faith. Give me the passion and zeal to do the works of Your kingdom and to run the race with my eyes set on You— the ultimate prize! In Jesus' name, Amen.

28

Endurance Sees

And so, after he had patiently endured,
he obtained the promise.
—Hebrews 6:15

an you stand the test of time? Endurance can be defined as the capacity to bear something unpleasant, painful, or difficult. It is also defined as suffering patiently. Christians can become weary of living in a debased world that's not compatible with holy lifestyles. Surely, Jesus experienced the extremity of these feelings, because He was a perfect light shining into a dark world, and the darkness could not comprehend Him. Rejection and sorrow were not absent from the Messiah's sentiments, but He didn't look back to His preexistent state in glory and gloomily compare it with His present condition, which was one of the extreme opposite. Rather, He looked to the result of His present condition. In other words, He looked to the future, the One "who for the joy that was set before him endured the cross, despising the shame, and is set down at the right hand of the throne of God" (Hebrews 12:2b).

As Christians, we are also aliens, strangers, and foreigners in a world led by the prince of the power of the air (Ephesians 2:2). Like Jesus, we can endure such contradiction, as we consider the joy that is set before us. In order to receive what God has for us we have to wait in patience. When the children of Israel were to destroy the enemy, the Lord didn't always send them out immediately. Rather, often He told them to "lie in wait." It takes patience to overcome the enemy and inherit the Promised Land. It takes time. Nevertheless, if you will endure and not turn back, but be persistent and patient, you shall gain the victory and possess the spoils! The Psalms stress that we are to wait upon the Lord, to be strong, and of good courage (Psalm 27:14). In the book of Isaiah, we find that those who wait on the Lord shall mount up with wings like eagles and soar.

But they that wait upon the LORD shall renew their strength; they shall mount up with wings as eagles; they shall run, and not be weary; and they shall walk, and not faint. — Isaiah 40:31

God has not left us without strong consolation. Abraham endured because he looked ahead. Jesus even said, "Your father Abraham rejoiced to see my day: and he saw it, and was glad" (John 8:56). Abraham believed the prophetic Word of the Lord and walked by faith and not by sight. He received the Word of the Lord concerning his inheritance, and with the prophecy, he fought a good fight of faith (Romans 4:20). Abraham's faith was strong because he embraced the Word and promises of God. Likewise, we are not to look at our present circumstances and stagger through unbelief, doubt, and discouragement. "A double minded man is unstable in all his ways" (James 1:8). Our circumstances do not define our identity, nor do they dictate our future. Rather, the Word of God defines our identity. God's promises define our future and tell us that we are not staying where we presently are, but can look forward to a greater tomorrow, as we surrender to God's will. This truth should solidify our commitment to the Lord and give us strength to be unmovable, abounding in the work of the Lord. This does not mean that we have never been lured by the affinity of carnality and fallen short of God's commandments, but it does mean that we are not giving up on our purpose and part in God's divine plan. Even when the enemy tries to snatch our hope for tomorrow right out of our present today, we are called to look upward to Him who holds the future. We just have to press onward and lay hold of the hope that is set before us regardless of our present circumstances.

Let us greatly consider the hope that is eternal because we have in heaven a better and an enduring substance (Hebrews 10:34).

If in this life only we have hope in Christ, we are of all men, most miserable.
— 1 Corinthians 15:19

Prayer

Father God, Creator of heaven and Earth, I pray for faith like Abraham to stand firm, to believe for things I can't see. Lord, I know that Your will for me is greater and more wonderful than anything I can imagine. I pray that I will forget the past and reach for the things ahead. Lord, give me strength to resist the tug of the world and a passion to press toward the mark for the prize of the high calling of God in Christ Jesus (Philippians 3:14).

29

Confidence Carries

For we are made partakers of Christ, if we hold the
beginning of our confidence stedfast unto the end;
—Hebrews 3:14

What does it mean to share in Christ or be a "partaker in Christ?" Does it not mean to partake of His life and His power, and to inherit His kingdom? How do we do it? We do it by casting not away our confidence in the Lord. Our confidence comes from our faith and trust in God. It is belief in the fact that God is who He says He is and that He will do what He says He will do. The children of Israel rejoiced in God's providence when they saw the Red Sea part, and they were delivered out of Egypt. What confidence they must have had in the Lord's provision and His protection. Imagine the display of their assurance in God as Miriam picked up the tambourine and the women followed her with tambourines and dancing (Exodus 15:20 NIV). And the children of Israel joined Moses in praising the Lord.

> Then sang Moses and the children of Israel this song unto the LORD, and spake, saying, I will sing unto the LORD, for he hath triumphed gloriously: the horse and his rider hath he thrown into the sea. — Exodus 15:1

They were truly confiding in God for their journey ahead, but they did not hold it steadfast until the end. Their confidence in God dwindled at the first stage of suffering. Instead of holding fast and looking to God for water to drink, they began to murmur and complain. God continued to do mighty miracles in the midst of them, and perhaps their trust was restored for a time. However, as soon as suffering came again, they lost their confidence in God's delivering power.

In Hebrews 3:8, the Lord beseeches us not to harden our hearts as in the provocation of the day of temptation in the wilderness. On that day, the children of Israel refused to go in and possess the land for fear of the enemy. It's easy to see that the less confident they were in the Lord, the more their hearts were hardened through unbelief toward God until, finally, they provoked Him to anger and the Lord swore in His wrath that they would not enter into

His rest (Psalm 95:11). God caused their carcasses to fall in the wilderness, and they did not enter the land because of unbelief. God allowed the children of Israel to go through the desolate wilderness to prove their hearts. He desired them to look unto Him for their water, food, shelter, and protection. For God had not left them hopeless. He revealed to them through Moses that their obedience would enable them to possess the land of hills and valleys that flows with milk and honey and that receives water from the rain of heaven. They knew that their obedience would cause showers of blessings to be upon them and their children. This included blessings on their land, store-houses, cattle, health, and more; so much so that the blessings would overtake them.

Nevertheless, they refused to endure the hard-ships in order to get to the Promised Land. Rather, they murmured, complained, and even looked back, desiring Egypt. All this came because they cast away their confidence in the Lord and ended up in unbelief. Our confidence in God is in believing and trusting in our hearts that His Word is true and, though we may not see His promises fulfilled in our lives yet, we know the fulfillment is coming! The promised future is coming! It's our confidence that carries us through the hard times in the wilderness on the way to possess the Promised Land.

Not all of the children of Israel forfeited the promises of God. Caleb said in bold assertion, "Let us go up at once, and possess it; for we are well able to overcome it" (Numbers 13:30b). Both Joshua and

Caleb confided in God and inherited their portions of the Promised Land.

Our confidence in God affirms our hope in God. For the Bible says hope is not seen. If we see it, then it's not hope (Romans 8:24). Hope has a future connotation to it. And our confidence in God keeps our hope for tomorrow alive. Though we may possess the promises of God today, we are hoping to possess even more tomorrow. The Bible exhorts us not to cast away our confidence, which has great recompense of reward (Hebrews 10:35). Though we suffer now, as long as we are trusting in God, we can rest assured our reward is coming! We can be confident of the blessing for this life and be assured of eternal life (1 John 2:25).

God desires for us to have a confidence that comes from Him. Confidence can be defined as a bold awareness that drives out all fear, worry, and anxiety. It is an unshakable assurance of God's faithfulness. In Philippians 4, we find that the basis for our confidence is the presence of the Lord, (v. 5) the peace of God, (v. 7) the strength of God (v. 13) and the promise of His provision (v. 19).

The ultimate ground of faith and knowledge is confidence in God.
—Charles Hodge 1894–1964

Prayer

Lord, Your Word says that it is better to trust in You than to put confidence in man (Psalm 118:8). Father, I pray I will not turn back, but press forward to the mark of the high call of God on my life. I pray that I will trust You, knowing that You are able to do exceedingly, abundantly above all that I ask or think according to the power of Jesus Christ that works in me (Ephesians 3:20). Amen.

30

Dreams Come True

*When the LORD turned again the captivity of Zion,
we were like them that dream. Then was our mouth
filled with laughter, and our tongue with singing:
then said they among the heathen, The LORD hath
done great things for them.*
—Psalm 126:1, 2

The dreams of the righteous come true, but the dreams of the ungodly will end (unfulfilled). The ungodly will seem like they are dreaming, but they will awaken and still be hungry and thirsty (Isaiah 29:8).

The God-given dreams of the righteous are too big for human hands to accomplish, but of course, not for God's hands. God given dreams give us hope for the future and remind us that we are destined for more than our present circumstances may indicate.

The children of Israel's dreams were attained when the Lord turned back their captivity. While in captivity, they wept by the rivers of Babylon as they remembered the blessing of Zion (Psalm 137:1). For seventy years, the exiled children of Israel prayed to return from Babylon to their beloved Jerusalem. But we discover in Psalm 126 that they saw their dreams become reality. They sowed in tears, but reaped in joy, as they joyfully exclaimed the fulfillment of the seemingly impossible, "The Lord hath done great things for us; whereof we are glad" (Psalm 126:3). They witnessed the phenomenon of the fulfillment of Jeremiah's prophesy; and lived out the excitement of returning to Jerusalem and rebuilding the Temple (Ezra 1:1–4).

God-given dreams are our impetus for pressing on towards a greater tomorrow, where we refuse to remain content with status quo. When we have dreams and aspirations from the Lord, we know that He is speaking and imparting the visions to us and as we live in obedience to Him, He makes impossibility possible. The spiritual revelation can soon become tangible. Recognizing the sovereign providence of God can remove the impediments from our expectations and deliver us from the selfish pride of thinking that we are in absolute control of our lives.

In addition to God-inspired dreams, we must be aware of worldly aspirations. Jesus taught about worldly goals in Luke 12, where He warned against all kinds of greed, and tells the story of the man who poured his life into building bigger barns to hoard his wealth. However, just as the man's egotistical dream was about to be realized, he died. His beauty turned to ashes and all he prepared for himself was a bed of judgment. Jesus taught us to be rich towards God (vv.15–21).

Dreams and visions are the essence of our lives and destinies. It's easy to stray from the Word of God when we don't keep His presence and promises near our hearts and before our eyes because "Where there is no vision, the people perish" (Proverbs 29:18).

Kingdom dreams and visions are not without opposition and persecution. Persecution will always come to those who live for the Lord (2 Timothy 3:12). Joseph brothers were jealous of his dreams because they didn't want him to excel or be exalted. In their eyes, he was just a spoiled younger brother and a ridiculous dreamer.

And they said one to another, Behold, this dreamer cometh. Come now therefore, and let us slay him, and cast him into some pit, and we will say, Some evil beast hath devoured him: and we shall see what will become of his dreams.—Genesis 37:19, 20

They wanted to kill him in order to kill his dreams. They already hated him because of his father's great love for him (Genesis 37:3), but for him to dream beyond the mediocre family traditions added injury to insult. How dare him to have God-given dreams that could challenge him to pursue a life beyond the status quo limitations of their tradition. This was outside the box of their manipulation and controlling family system. The only solution in their eyes was to strip him of his garments, cast him into a pit, and sell him to slavery.

However, the same God who imparted the dreams was faithful to fulfill them, as Joseph remained obedient. Joseph's dreams came true. He was exalted over Egypt and saw his brothers bow down before him and was instrumental in saving their lives, along with many others. Contrary to worldly aspirations, kingdom dreams are not all about us, but include the fulfillment of destiny for others as well. It is so encouraging to know that God allows His devout followers to see the fulfillment of the passions and desires that He has birthed and to know that it's for a reason that's greater than we can fathom! Whether we see our dreams fulfilled now or later, we should not become weary in well doing. We must believe that God's prophecies will come to pass, and we simply have to fight a good fight of faith with the word of prophecy. We need to be like Jacob and keep envisioning the ladder of ascent, which comes through humility, endurance, and confidence.

Trust God to give you only the dreams that matter. Dreams from God are about purpose and destiny — they are big and bold. God is calling you to dream. Dare to dream big, refusing to be content with status quo. Dare to dream bold, refusing to conform to other's manipulated agendas. Dare to dream for God because we have an awesome God who is more than able to impart and fulfill them.

Expect great things from God; attempt great things for God.
—William Carey

Prayer

Lord, I thank You for prophetic dreams and visions that You have given me and the new ones You are going to birth. Lord, I believe Your Word is true and it will not return void (Isaiah 55:11). I believe if You spoke it, You will do it and if You said it, You will bring it to pass (Numbers 23:18). Lord, let all flesh be silent and let Your Word stand above all voices and opinions of others. Father, I pray that I will not grow weary in well doing, but will be steadfast, unmovable always abounding in Your work (1 Corinthians 15:58). In Jesus' name. Amen.

Part 8
The Last Cry

31

Soul Travail

Behold, the righteous shall be recompensed in the earth: much more the wicked and the sinner.
—Proverbs 11:31

Even though the world rejoices, it will also lament. The disobedient can be described as barren, but will ironically experience birth pangs:

For when they shall say, Peace and safety; then sudden destruction cometh upon them, as travail upon a woman with child; and they shall not escape.—1 Thessalonians 5:3

Just as when Israel was living in disobedience to the Lord, pains came upon the priest's daughter-in-law and her time to give birth was also the time of her death; so it shall be for the disobedient. They will suffer travail and bring forth Ichabod (the glory has departed). Both believers and unbelievers will experience birth pangs in these last days.

The closer we get to the fulfillment of prophesy and the coming of the Lord, the more intense and rapid the birth pangs will become. But it is far more rewarding and glorious to "labor" for righteousness than with the cries of destruction.

The Bride of Christ is an antitype of Mary, who gave birth to the Messiah. While Simeon blessed the parents of Jesus, he said to Mary, "(Yea, a sword shall pierce through thy own soul also,)" (Luke 2:35). Again we see the Kingdom Principle: included in the blessing was the prerequisite to suffer. Mary herself said, "for, behold, from henceforth all generations shall call me blessed" (Luke 1:48). But this did not change the fact that her name, Miriam, came from the Hebrew root word *Marah*, which means *bitter*. However, through the Messiah, her bitter would become sweet. In the book of Exodus we learn that God told Moses to cast a tree into the bitter waters of Marah to turn them sweet (15:24). As for Jesus' mother, there was a bitter piercing of her soul as she saw her son slain upon the cruel cross, but the cross was also the "tree" that turned her bitter pain into sweet salvation.

Likewise, with Christ, we experience bitter agony for a season, but the cross is also the tree that turns our bitter pain eternally sweet. As we pick up our cross and follow Him, we become impregnated with a passion to birth His kingdom in these last days. Jesus told His disciples:

Verily, verily, I say unto you, That ye shall weep and lament, but the world shall rejoice: and ye shall be sorrowful, but your sorrow shall be turned into joy. A woman when she is in travail hath sorrow, because her hour is come: but as soon as she is delivered of the child, she remembereth no more the anguish, for joy that a man is born into the world.

—John 16:20, 21

Even as Mary was a virgin when she birthed the Messiah, so the Bride of Christ is a spiritual virgin daughter of Zion called to birth forth the Messiah's return. "Therefore the Lord himself shall give you a sign; Behold, a virgin shall conceive, and bear a son, and shall call his name Immanuel" (Isaiah 7:14). As the Messiah is birthed through the travail of Zion, God is establishing His kingdom upon the throne of David.

For unto us a child is born, unto us a son is given: and the government shall be upon his shoulder: and his name shall be called Wonderful, Counseller, The mighty God, The everlasting Father, The Prince of Peace. Of the increase of his government and peace there shall be no end, upon the throne of David, and upon his kingdom, to order it, and to establish it with judgment and with justice from henceforth even for ever. The zeal of the LORD of hosts will perform this.

—Isaiah 9:6, 7

The sanctified Bride of Christ is birthing forth the Messiah, through pangs of passion and travail, in these last days. Travail is painful or toilsome work and can involve the physical and the mental. The Hebrew words for "travail" mean misery, trouble and sorrow. Travail frequently carries meanings associated with childbirth such as: deliver, bear, pain and bring forth. Travailing in the Spirit is intense prayer and intercession, accompanied with inward agony and pain, to birth spiritual passions and pursuits. This is exemplified in the woman prophesied in the book of Revelation:

And she being with child cried, travailing in birth, and pained to be delivered...And she brought forth a man child, who was to rule all nations with a rod of iron: and her child was caught up unto God, and to his throne. — Revelation 12:2-5

It is the ones who suffer with Jesus and birth His kingdom on the earth that will reign with Him upon His throne. "If we suffer, we shall also reign with him" (2 Timothy 2:12a). It was the travail of Jesus' soul that birthed us into His kingdom; likewise, it is the travail of the saints that is birthing Him and the fullness of His kingdom in the earth. This painstaking cry has been echoing throughout the earth for millenniums, but in these last days it is growing louder and louder.

There may be weeping for a night, but joy comes in the morning (Psalm 30:5). For Isaiah prophesied that the Messiah would see the travail of His soul: "He shall see of the travail of his soul, and shall be satisfied" (53:11a). As Jesus will see the full results of the travail of His soul, so will the Bride of Christ see the impact of the travail of her soul and the reward thereof. Our pain is not in vain. Don't dare turn back now because the reward is still on the way.

Behold, the LORD hath proclaimed unto the end of the world, Say ye to the daughter of Zion, Behold, thy salvation cometh; behold, his reward is with him, and his work before him. And they shall call them, The holy people, The redeemed of the LORD: and thou shalt be called, Sought out, A city not forsaken. —Isaiah 62:11, 12

As the Messiah's glory is revealed, so is the glory of the Bride. We, who receive the prophet Jesus, in His name, shall receive His reward. And we who receive the righteous man Jesus, in His name, shall receive His reward (Matthew 10:41). Thus it is the Bride who shares in the spoils and the inheritance. The sufferings are nothing compared with the hundredfold return and the eternal glory that shall be revealed in the Bride of Christ.

For our light affliction, which is but for a moment, worketh for us a far more exceeding and eternal weight of glory;
                              —2 Corinthians 4:17

The time will come when those who have suffered with Him shall no more remember their anguish, but will rejoice and have joy that no one can take away (John 16:22).

Shall I bring to the birth, and not cause to bring forth? saith the LORD: shall I cause to bring forth, and shut the womb? saith thy God. Rejoice ye with Jerusalem, and be glad with her, all ye that love her: rejoice for joy with her, all ye that mourn for her:
—Isaiah 66:9, 10

Prayer

Father, I am crying out for You to manifest Your kingdom in this earth. The Spirit and the Bride, we cry out to You to come quickly. Lord, we long for Your presence and power. We want more — more of You Lord.

32

The Ultimate Suffering

*The fear of the LORD is clean, enduring for ever:
the judgments of the LORD are true and righteous
altogether. More to be desired are they than gold,
yea, than much fine gold: sweeter also than honey
and the honeycomb. Moreover by them is thy
servant warned: and in keeping of
them there is great reward.*
—Psalm 19:9–11

John the Revelator wept much because no man in
heaven, nor on the earth, nor under the earth, nor
in the sea was worthy to open the book and to loose its
seals (Revelation 5:2-4). But the seals would unleash
horrific judgments upon the wicked, so why would
John have such a desire for the book to be opened
that he would weep? He passionately desired to see

God's kingdom manifest in the earth. Consequently, the wicked are judged and the righteous reign in the righteousness of Christ as kings and priests.

The ultimate suffering has never and will never be experienced by Christians. Martyrs who are brutally and excruciatingly tortured do not experience the ultimate pain. Christians who experience an agonizing death, regardless of the cause, do not taste the greatest strength of death's sting. Even as God raised Jesus, the pains of death were loosed because Jesus could not be held by death (Acts 2:24). Likewise, they are loosed for all who believe on Him because neither can the pains of death hold God's children.

Jesus said, "I am the resurrection, and the life: he that believeth in me, though he were dead, yet shall he live" (John 11:25). It was through death that Jesus destroyed him who had the power of death; that is, the devil. Scripture reveals that the sting of death is sin (1 Corinthians 15:56). The sting has caused men to be in bondage all their lives to the dread of death. But Jesus delivered us from sin, the sting of death and its fear and torment, "And deliver them who through fear of death were all their lifetime subject to bondage" (Hebrews 2:15). Some may argue that Christians aren't delivered from death because mortal bodies still decease.

However, Christians are delivered from death's staunch eternal hold and are liberated through death from mortality to immortality—"Thou fool, that which thou sowest is not quickened, except it die" (1 Corinthians 15:36). How glorious it must be to be transferred to a place free from death, sorrow, crying, and pain. Moreover, yes, death will ultimately be destroyed (1 Corinthians 15:26). It will be swallowed up in victory. For it is written,

O death, where is thy sting? O grave, where is thy victory...But thanks be to God, which giveth us the victory through our Lord Jesus Christ! — 1 Corinthians 15:55-55

Satan and his cohorts are the ones who will experience the ultimate pain. They know this, and that is why the demons cried out to Jesus, saying, "'What have we to do with thee, Jesus, thou Son of God? art thou come hither to torment us before the time?'" (Matthew 8:29). The unrepentant will share in Satan's portion of suffering. For the Bible says that the wicked will be cast into outer darkness and there shall be weeping and gnashing of teeth (Matthew 8:12). Jesus also said that the wicked will be thrown into a furnace of fire (Matthew 13:42).

In the book of Revelation, we find that the sting of demonic powers will be so strong and the torment so great that the wicked will desire death.

And in those days shall men seek death, and shall not find it; and shall desire to die, and death shall flee from them.

—Revelation 9:6

The sorrows of death and the pains of hell will encompass and take hold of them, but they will not be loosed from the torment. The greatest pain will be experienced by the devil, the beast, the false prophet, death and hell and whosoever's name is not found written in the Book of Life. They will be tormented day and night forever and ever (Revelation 20:10).

But for the redeemed of the Lord, the day will come when the cry of anguish will never be heard again, hearts will never be broken again, no tear will ever again flow from the eye, and death will be unknown! The final judgment condemns these things to the lake of fire.

The word *mourning* or *sorrow* in the Greek text, *penyov*, denotes sorrow or grief of any kind. This includes sorrow for the loss of property, friends, or loved ones; sorrow for disappointment, persecution, sickness; sorrow for sin or disobedience. Imagine a world where there is no sorrow, no grief, no persecution, no abuse, and no fear. Imagine a place that's sinless: painless, tearless, and deathless. What a great recompense of reward that's worth living and dying for!

*And God shall wipe away all tears from their eyes;
and there shall be no more death, neither sorrow,
nor crying, neither shall there be any more pain: for
the former things are passed away.*
—Revelation 21:4.

Prayer

O' Lord—what a day of rejoicing that will be—
when I see You, I see Your face, I gaze into Your
beautiful eyes, and instantly, all pain disappears, and
pure joy permeates every ounce of my being. I thank
You so much for dying for me! I thank You so much
for Victory! I thank You so much, sweet Jesus, for
loving me. Use me anyway You want Lord. I'm all
Yours. Amen.

Printed in the United States
204043BV00001B/82-366/A

9 781602 661271